"It is towards the future that we have labored with these concepts, to make them understandable, workable and tremendously effective. We hope others will seize this work and blaze a new pathway that does not use the old and barren promotional approaches" —Paul Snyder

ANALYZING, INTERPRETING AND UNDERSTANDING THE MEDICAL LITERATURE©

I0480143

A GUIDE FOR THE PHARMACEUTICAL REPRESENTATIVE, PHARMD, NP AND PA

WITH SPECIAL EMPHASIS ON:

- Using medical studies to gain market share---advanced course

- Learning how to spot "BIAS" in a study

- Understanding how to dissect and interpret the "Material & Method" section of a journal study

- Knowing how to present and discuss journal articles

- Learning how to understand and discuss "half-life", "area under the curve" and "p-value"

- Finding the answers to *"The Who"* questions in a study---
  - Who wrote study design?
  - Who decided sample size?
  - Who verified testing, randomization & blinding?
  - Who chose the methods used in arms of study?
  - Who summarized retrospective studies?

- Questions clinicians ask about studies

- Sample Sales Presentations Using A Medical Journal Study---First Encounter and 30-Second Stand-Up

BY

SHEELEY CONSULTING GROUP, LLC

Consulting: Sales: Marketing: Advertising: Management: publications

Presented as part of Sheeley Consulting Group
Clinical Study Analysis Program

Published by:

A Book's Mind

PO Box 272847

Fort Collins, CO 80527

Copyright © 2019 Sheeley Consulting LLC. All Rights Reserved.

ISBN: 978-1-949563-62-7

Printed in the United States of America

ACKNOWLEDGMENTS

Paul and I are grateful to the many friends of distinction who have contributed to the content and writing of this book and the other two books we have written. In particular, special thanks to my daughter Stacy who helped us find Brian Dunne the best website design guy on this planet, and for all her ideas on layout design and content.

I would also like to give thanks to Dave Beckwith, Mike Monti , Ann Grana, Peter Bornstein and Henry Trenkle for their insightful comments, suggestions, and editing work. To Charley McLeskey, MD, Astra Zeneca, for his years of friendship and for his ideas on what title to give each book. Thank you to my wife, Diane, for her sage advice with this book. To Floyd Orfield and his team at "*A Book's Mind*" for cover design, and publishing, they are the best in the business. These books could not have been written alone by either Paul or me…it was the synergy between us that captured all of these concepts and made them understandable. As Paul said, *"we hope others will seize this work and blaze a new pathway that does not use the old and barren promotional approaches."* We hope you do. It was a great, once-in-a-lifetime opportunity to work with Paul in writing these three books…he is truly a genius in the pharmaceutical arena.

FOREWORD

"The years teach much which the days never knew" —Ralph Waldo Emerson

We dedicate this Manual to all the pharmaceutical Representatives we worked with, supervised and competed against. It was the competition from Eli Lilly, Bristol-Meyers Squibb, Pfizer, Merck, and McNeil that really got us very interested in understanding how to break down and dissect a medical journal article. They were using medical studies against us, and to survive, we had to learn and adjust quickly. And the physicians at the major teaching hospitals, (Washington U School of Medicine in St Louis---Barnes-Jewish Hospital), weren't going to be sold using the literature we were using.

When I was promoted to teaching hospital representative calling on Washington University, St Louis University and the University of Missouri Medical Center in Columbia, MO, my days of using the *"Madison Avenue"* glossy literature the company provided were long gone. I shudder to think my showing the Chief of Urology, Barnes Hospital in St Louis, MO a piece of *"Madison Avenue"* literature showing the benefits of our antibiotic in UTIs.

We spent a lot of time gaining permission to attend Grand Rounds programs and Journal Club meetings to hear how physicians themselves dissected a medical study and, equally important, how they think and presented the study. We figured if we were going to present a study to a provider, we would need to know what to present in the study. And. as we learned, there are a small number of books written on the different parts (abstract, introduction, material & methods, results, etc) of a medical study, but we could not find any book on how to present a study whether you have plenty of time to do so with a provider or have only 30-seconds to present.

So we developed our own medical study *"**Viral Elimination In Humans**"* in the ***"United States Journal of Medicine"*** to show our readers how we would present this study at a Grand Rounds program.

We think most representatives stayed clear of presenting medical studies approved by their company because of the fear they would not be able to answer the questions providers would ask. And, most likely, their Sales Training Department, during their basic training classes never taught them how to break down and present a medical study. Basic Training, for me, included a week of how to sell pharmaceuticals patterned after the Xerox Professional Selling Skills course. We didn't sell copy machines, but we were learning how Xerox sold copy machines hoping that what we learned would be the best way to sell a physician to use Actifed, for example. We did not feel the Xerox approach was effective because the course was a *"tell-tell-tell-close"* approach.

I think most representatives, if they were being honest, felt the same way about the Xerox Professional Selling Skills course as we did. And, it was this course which led to so much   frustration within the representative staff. Frustration is one thing, but loss of sales was another, and when they started losing business to the competition, who had incorporated medical studies into their presentations, they reverted to the only thing they knew. Sell on personality and whether you deserved or earned the right to ask the provider to use your product, the close became paramount.

The more business lost, the close, which stated out with *"doctor, would you use a little of my stuff*, graduated into grilling the provider on why he wasn't using *"my stuff"*. Inexperienced District Sales Managers, accompanying a representative on a sales call, began to get into the act and pressure the doctor even more as to why he was not using their product. So it was only natural that doctors began to shut their doors to sales representatives, and, many to District Managers as well.

Doctors closed their doors not only because of the pressure being applied by representative who thought they were selling used cars, but because the representatives, using Xerox sales techniques, offered nothing of value to the provider at a time when a provider was getting more and more pressed for time. Back in the day, the physicians in the *"country"* portion of my territory as a representative calling on office-based providers, would spend 20-minutes with me in their office.

Several sales representatives and District Sales Managers are going to look at this Manual as *"nice-to-know"* because their company will not allow them to use medical studies in their presentations. I would say this is the wrong approach for the following reasons. First, understanding a study about one of your products, or your competitor's products, would result in much greater confidence and job satisfaction. What if you are making a sales call and a provider asks about a new study with one of your products. While you can't answer any questions about the study, you are thoroughly aware of the study. Another reason for knowing how to analyze a medical study is to better understand your promotional marketing background and insight into the way your marketing and sales points were clinically studied. This background provides deep understanding of how your marketing points were actually extracted from your clinical studies, and the studies of your competitor's as well.

We know by reading and re-reading this Manual you will benefit a great deal. We encourage you to obtain permission to attend Grand Rounds programs and Journal Club meetings. Listen to how a study is presented and learn how providers think. We encourage you to spend some time with the section of this Manual which outlines how we would present the *United States Journal of Medicine* study at a Grand Rounds presentation or Journal Club.

Lastly, we wish to call to your attention a book Paul Snyder and I wrote entitled ***"How To Sell Pharmaceuticals & Medical Devices When You Are Really Not Sure How"***. If you are stuck in the *"tell-tell-tell-close"* or *"fact-fact-fact-close"* sales presentation method, this book is a must read. It isn't a big book and we think it is dynamic because it teaches you how to move beyond the *"tell-tell-tell-close"* sales method.

Most importantly, this book will teach you the concept of *"**Patient-Type Centered** Selling©* which you can incorporate into your approved sales promotional selling pieces. There is one other thing this book teaches you that is worth its weight in gold and that is how to get a provider to use your product for the first time. And, wouldn't it be more than nice to know that when you call on one of the providers in your territory that you know and understand how he was trained to think and make drug selection decisions.

There is no sales program in all of pharma that will teach you how providers think and how they select the drugs they do. Because if you know how a provider thinks, you know how to present your product in a manner that makes sense. And, there is no sales program that teaches you how to get a provider to use your drug for the first time. In our opinion, getting a physician to use your drug for the first time is the most difficult challenge of all. This book teaches both.

We welcome your comments and questions…let us hear from you.

Ron Sheeley
Rsheeley09@gmail.com

Paul Snyder
Psnyder1@indy.rr.com

It ain't what you don't know that will get you in trouble. It is what you know
for sure that just ain't so" —Mark Twain

INTRODUCTION

Of all the tools available to market medical products based upon scientific study, the clinical study or medical journal article provides the best source to present information in a manner in which clinicians have been trained to think, understand and make treatment selection decisions. Sheeley Consulting can apply their insights in many different arenas, such as creating advertising/marketing pieces, working with PharmD's and Medical liaisons, or schools for NP's, PA's to name a few.

Our Basic Premise:

Throughout medical school, internships and residencies, clinicians learn to review and discuss medical journal articles. At grand rounds programs, journal club meetings and specialty team conferences, clinical studies are dissected and discussed. Once in practice, clinicians rely on these resources not only to keep up-to-date, but also to consider how the evidence in studies can be implemented into their daily practices. Collectively, these resources can drive changes in guidelines and "best practices" through what is called *"evidence-based medicine"* (EBM).

The Challenge Today: Time is at a premium

There are so many General-focus journals and Specialty journals publishing studies that clinicians are challenged in two ways: First, how does one find out what is important enough to consider? Second, how does one find the time to read even the abstracts of those studies when there is great pressure to manage more patients in even shorter treatment room visits?

Medical studies are produced with the goal of answering questions to improve patient outcome or quality of life. Their proposition is to insert change into or modify treatment regimens. In producing treatment change, a question of 'time invested to yield change-inducing results' is the challenge.

Following that hindrance is one of creating a specific patient to represent the thought before adding new insight into memory. Merely adding numerical result-oriented data to memorize is a slow process and requires a jump from data to patient treatment changes. Certainly, there is no better source than Medical Journal articles. Our tools enable you to bring quick, interesting aspects to your clinicians, quickly acknowledging that time invested needs to be as short as possible while maximizing usefulness to specific patients.

Make data helpful for specific patients

We have observed through the years that the outstanding presenters knew how to read, dissect, understand, and most importantly, use journal articles to make patient-specific points. These insights work in a wide variety of situations and scenarios.

This guide/manual is all about knowing how to use, evaluate and read a wide variety of journal articles. Because when it gets right down to it, clinicians are trained to make decisions based on information that they get at conferences, grand rounds programs, journal-club meetings, speaker-dinner meetings, etc. Information presented to them that appears in current and older medical journal articles. The key point is that data itself is not a patient. We want to shorten or eliminate the mental question of *"how would that patient present when I walk into the room?'*

TO HELP YOU *"LEARN MORE ABOUT IT"* WE HAVE PROVIDED YOU WITH:

- **A Sample Journal Study/Reprint** This "sample" "*United States Journal of Medicine*" "*Viral Elimination in Humans*" reprint is will show you where the sections are that are being discussed, and to give real meaning to the 2-case scenarios we provide.

- **"*Unites States Journal of Medicine*" (sample journal study)**

  - **Review Questions**

  - **Study Guide and Representative Goals**

  - **Manager Guide**

  - **Two Case Studies**

- **Guide to Reprints**. A review of a reprint, section by section, from the point of view of a presenter of clinical data who has the task of making the data come alive.

- ***Nota Bene*** (*Latin:observe carefully*) – Our tips about how you can apply the learning to make an impact and improve patient outcome or quality of life.

- **Briefing Guide**. A guide to writing up your own article briefs to position for the presentation. [This Guide can also be used as a post-test or as part of a group learning activity.]

- **A Complete Review Of How to Spot Bias in a Clinical Study**

"It is not that I'm so smart, it is just that I stay with a problem longer" —Albert Einstein

OVERVIEW:
FROM CLINICAL STUDY TO PRESENTATION

If there is anything that leads clinicians modify their approach, it is an insightful new Clinical Study. It may be academically interesting, but if it is not useful and memorable, little has been accomplished.

QUESTIONS CLINICIANS USUALLY ASK ABOUT STUDIES

From conducting in-depth interviews with teaching hospital and office-based sales approaches, we have learned that one of the major reasons clinicians do not like to encounter medical journal articles is that the points made are less than memorable and often not significant to their practice.

Let's say you have an approved journal article that compares your approach to a present practice of patient treatment. The results appearing in the article show that your approach is superior to an established therapy. The study is multi-centered, double-blinded, and placebo-controlled. The authors are experts in their field. You want to design a promotion with charts and graphs which are certainly better than columns of figures.

Because you want to highlight results in presenting a journal article, the majority of questions from clinicians arise as to how the results of the study compared and how the results were obtained.

Here are some of the **questions you can anticipate** in selecting data from the paper described above:

- How did the results of your approach compare with the results of the established regimen?

- What key points are in the *Materials and Methods* section?

- Where was the study done?

- Who supported the study?

- Authors?

- How many patients participated in the study?

- Patient population---what patient types were included? Excluded?

- How was the study designed?

- What untoward effects were observed?

- What regimen was used?

Using the reprint ("*The United States Journal of Medicine*") we have supplied as a guide, we'll walk you through a reprint so you can answer all these questions from your clinicians with confidence.

And more importantly, our approach will yield greater acceptance and a higher regard for the presentation.

"Give a mall boy a hammer and he will find that everything he encounters needs pounding" —Kaplan's Law

HOW TO APPROACH A MEDICAL JOURNAL ARTICLE

A journal article is just like any other type of formal communication. It has a certain structure that it follows to make it easier for its audience to follow and find the information they seek. For instance, in a movie, you expect the credits to be at the end, with the starring roles at the front. In a journal article, the same holds true. The stars (the authors) are listed right under the title. If there were many physicians involved in the study reported, they are listed at the end. So are the references. But, in a movie, you don't expect the ending to be told up front. And you don't expect a summary of the story. In a journal article, that is exactly the expectation. In a journal article, this is what is called *"The Abstract"*.

Most clinicians 'read' many journal articles by scanning the abstracts. This leaves the abstract section of the paper as the only part actually 'read". Since it is usually a short statement of the goal and results of the study, most physicians will only take the time to look at the results. Because of this, it is important for you to be able to tell the rest of the story, and understand why the study was initiated in the first place, what the results are and what they mean to specific patients in your daily practices.

Treaters want rapid, accurate answers to their questions, and you are investing your time to bring them a polished presentation by having thoroughly read, re-read and digested any reprint you have been given by the company.

So, when you look at a journal article, review all its parts:

- The Authors

- The Abstract

- The Introduction

- Materials and Methods

- Results

- Discussion

- References

Some areas have more weight than others, but all have value. Using the reprint supplied for reference, here's a Guide to get you on the road:

AUTHORS

Never underestimate the *"who"* value of an article. Look at the names of the authors and their institutions. In every specialty, there are nationally recognized experts. Getting to know their names helps you in determining how much credence or weight a particular study might carry.

Look also to see if there are disclosures about funding or corporate ties. This will either be listed up front under the authors, or at the end of the article. Currently, all funding or affiliation with industry MUST be listed somewhere in the paper, to address any financial bias.

THE ABSTRACT

The abstract appears under the title of the paper, and usually contains the following sections:

- **Content**. Gives the overview of where the paper is designed to fit.

- **Objective.** Outlines what the authors wanted to do.

- **Design.** How the study was planned and conducted. Double-blinded, randomized, place-bo-controlled trials are very good. They mean the researchers did not know what drug they were giving each patient (blinded); if patients were given drug (placebo-control, random-ized) and they noted progress by charting changes after patient visits (double-blinded). Setting, or where the study was conducted can be interesting. Multiple sites are more likely to eliminate the chance that a single institution had a procedure that was unusual. On the other hand, it is harder to control variables when the study was done at many sites.

- **Participants.** Tells how many patients were initially entered into the study. The notation *"n=976"* means 976 patients were in that part of the study. When a physician asks, "what is the *'n'?"* this is what they want to know---the total number of patients entered. Larger numbers generally support stronger results.

- **Intervention.** Tells what was administered and the criteria for using the treatment or approach.

- **Main Outcome Measures**. The endpoints that were used to determine the results of the study. Results are important because this section is one that doctors read. The validity of the study results, or "*p* value" will also be found here. This will tell you if the results are significant or not. Authors determine the cutoff points to demonstrate p-value.

- **Conclusion.** A summary of the key finding.

Nota Bene

This section of a journal article is most widely read by physicians. It outlines the goal of the study, the study results and a sentence or two on the final conclusion. Think of the abstract as a highlights reel. It is a condensed version of the rest of the whole game. From a presenter's perspective, when a clinician reads only the abstract, s/he only gets the highlights. So you need to acknowledge both parts: the highlights reel (the Abstract) and the whole game (the rest of the paper, mostly notably the Materials and Methods section). Rarely are insights or patient descriptions included, which are key points.

INTRODUCTION

This section presents information on why the authors wrote the paper in the first place, states background comments and usually briefly outlines past written work on the subject. The introductory section provides you with some very good 'insight' on how to open up a discussion of a paper with your audience. This is the "*why bother?*" part of the paper. If the authors cannot show this study is important, it usually will not be published in a respected, peer-reviewed journal.

THE "MATERIALS & METHODS" SECTION: THE HEART OF THE MATTER

While the vast majority of physicians only have time to read the Abstract section of an article/study, the section you want to study first is the *"Materials & Methods"* section. The Materials & Methods provides the heartbeat of the paper.

When it comes to discussing an article with an audience, if a question is asked, the question usually refers to how the study was designed. This is not found in the Abstract or Discussion Section. It is found here, in the Materials and Methods.

Understanding this section takes more time, and that effort will really set you apart from *'the pack'* of presenters. It is a hard slog if you are not familiar with the terms, but it is worth it. Study design and methods are critical to the conclusions, as they can prove or disprove the hypothesis or reason for the study. A poor design means poor results, or results that are suspect. For the researcher/author, this is the most important part of the paper. It allows the author to make a valid point, acceptable to their colleagues and the scientific community. Knowing it makes your product a valuable resource.

Nota Bene

Put your self in a Treater's position…if you only have time to read abstracts and a presenter presents the results of a study [in a vacuum], without knowing how the study was designed, who would you listen to, the presenter who outlines study design and can use the study in context before presenting results or a presenter or product that just presents a chart showing 90% efficacy according to so and so's study?

There are many different terms used to describe study designs. We have listed most common under **"Factors Determining Study Design"** and more may be found in the **"Terms you need to know"** section].

For your presentation/promotion the key is not to get lost in the sea of study design terminology but to understand and be able to identify how studies are put together and structured. Did the plan make sense? Is it providing information that is repeatable in every day experience, or something only a physician with a lab at immediate call and patient's with large bank accounts can use?

Checking out the design will assist you in analyzing the methods used, the results obtained and the comments made within the article relative to validity.

Nota Bene

When you break down a study, it is often helpful to Map Out the design. Most of us remember better when we can "*see*" how something works.

The *"Who"* questions about the fine points of clinical studies:

- **Who came up with the study hypothesis**?

  This question relates in part to the disclosure of any affiliations of researchers with the manu-facturers/products being utilized. Further, is the hypothesis one that can clearly add clarity to deciding among present approaches with risk versus benefit?

  Carrying out a prospective clinical study is both very expensive and time consuming with much attention to detail. People design the studies, and thus they bring their own beliefs with them that can be unintentionally yield study bias. How controlled the data collection portion is can reduce some of the interviewing bias. This is important when positive and negative patient impressions are recorded.

- **Who chose the methods or products used in the arms of the study?**

  Often early studies are comparing a new product with placebo. Later, other current approaches may be included in further studies.

  If the choices were among the best current therapeutic approaches, what aspects of therapy did the study design include? If the other arm of the study is occupied by a product with a fairly high rate of a particular side effect or less than desired efficacy, was it chosen to enhance the clinical results of the new approach?

- **Who wrote the design of the study?**

  An important aspect is to look closely at the starting number=('n') of patients enrolled, and what number of patients were dropped, lost, or eliminated from the study data.

  The design likely includes what data will be collected about each patient, and what testing will be done to assure safety, efficacy, and untoward effects.

     □   Is there a point where the codes may be broken to determine if an early end to the study is warranted either due to unexpected efficacy or side effects?

     □   Were the enrolled patients grouped to include coverage of ages, sexes, and study entry clinical and laboratory status?

     □   If patients were chosen to most likely yield a positive outcome to the studied approach, how can a clinician use the data to likely help individual patients?

Importantly, since most patient populations yield a bell-shaped distribution curve, if a group of patients on the smaller flanges of the distribution curve are eliminated, valuable comparative data may be unintentionally overlooked. Additionally, there are a number of concerns about why a group of patients may be reported as 'lost to follow-up'. This has been referred to as '*biased attrition*'. If an interim analysis is part of the study, results may be so compelling that intervention or stopping the study happens.

- **Who decided the sample size?**

Determining how many patients to enroll is vital to achieve a valid outcome. Larger numbers reduce the chance of a sequence of patients with unanticipated outcomes or side effects affecting the overall results of the study.

That is why knowing clinicians ask what the "n" number is, so they can mentally see how memorable the results were. With small numbers, it is all too easy to assume outcomes that 'after this, therefore because of this' show efficacy. This is confusing to the public as advertising gives single examples of single uses that 'remove all stains immediately'. Thus, the general public has extreme challenges in understanding well designed clinical studies.

- **Who verified the testing, randomization and blinding?**

Investigational review boards verify much of this data, though it is critical that these aspects are controlled so that outcomes are not based upon preconceived philosophy. When more than one institution is involved to obtain greater patient enrollment numbers, it becomes challenging to have the same controls utilized at each institution.

The question of consistent patient chart review is very hard to verify. There are standards for reporting diagnostic accuracy, called STARD, though diagnostic tests change, and *methods can vary between institutions*. Subjective aspects such as patient quality of life are among the more difficult findings to evaluate. Tests have three aspects – *Sensitivity* to prove the disease, *Specificity* to identify those without the disease, and *predictive value* to find false positives and negatives. An increasingly important aspect of testing is the cost versus benefit or efficacy of the test, sometimes referred to as '*bang for the buck*', while trying to narrow a differential diagnosis.

- **Who summarized the <u>retrospective studies</u>?**

This point and the following one relate to studies that attempt to look at all past studies that relate to a particular clinical diagnosis or approach. The pooling of data to increase sample size may be attempted.

One value of a study that looks at all previous published papers is that it can help clinicians come to a consensus approach based upon past experience. The challenge in looking at earlier studies is that they very rarely have the same enrollment, testing and screening. Testing methods continue to be improved, and thus earlier results are very difficult to exactly compare.

For these reasons, retrospective studies are felt to have less clinical relevance than well designed, focused individual studies. Treatment parameters change over time so that intent to treat can render two studies done at different times very daunting to compare. The same is true of outcome measures as they also are modified over time. There have been a number of retrospective studies published, and the time spent to collect the published data is large indeed. General impressions may be the best aspect of these studies.

Prospective studies look forward, for example proposing further studies on a patient group to examine longer-term patient outcomes.

Importantly, never should only a selected few studies be selected apart from the long list of those collected retrospectively.

- **Who verified the interpretation of extracted data from <u>retrospective studies</u>?**

This key point requires a lot of clinical experience to assist in obtaining an overview of a number of different earlier approaches. Each paper cited needs to be analyzed to see how the designs and testing differed, and how each study established risk versus benefit in patient outcomes.

It is a challenge to focus on the entire body of studies and not extract one or two more favorable outcomes and imply that all the rest agree. The interpretation of data from all studies also needs to look at enrolled patient data that includes demographics and diagnostic findings.

- **Who collects the data? How is it handled?**

The amount of data generated by a clinical study is expensive, large in volume and complex. Patients can be lost to follow up, and any blinding must be maintained so that both patient and clinician are unaware of actual product or approach used. Thus, the data upon entry, during the study, and at the end are very crucial and sensitive. Study monitoring individuals often oversee this data for accuracy and security.

- **Who monitored the abstract, choosing the points of emphasis?**

It is a true challenge to compose an abstract so that everything is summarized without undue emphasis on one aspect. The intent of the study is noted, along with patient numbers and outcomes and demographics. The details are found later in the paper.

- **Who chooses the 250 words to remain in a truncated abstract?**

Often this shortened version is all that busy clinicians have time to read. Journals may publish abstracts from other Medical journals that relate to a particular specialty.

Medline searches can truncate the abstracts at 250 words. Many abstracts are much longer than that limit, so some information that might be insightful to a clinician will remain within the study itself.   Clinicians have told us many times that "they read the paper" though it is only the abstract they have time for unless they are preparing a patient for presentation to specialty or general rounds during residency.

Also, medical centers and specialty groups may have more advanced testing and imaging than community hospitals and family practices so it can be a difficult task to compare sites in a multi-center study. Hopefully the methods and tests used are practical in nature with lower costs involved.

Control groups have been a standard comparative part of studies. It is important to look at how these groups compare to the treatment group as variables can vastly affect the validity of the data. The difficulty of finding matching paired populations is very hard to guarantee.

Using Random selection to create paired treatment and observation populations is a good way to reduce selectin bias.

Then comes a pair of terms that relate to the question of practicality – *reliability* and *validity*, and that question can be answered scientifically by a second study to see if the results are reproducible.

Distribution calculations or measurements – graphing sites on the curve: The *mean* point is adding values and dividing by how many values were added. It will not be the highest or the middle. (If *standard deviation* is calculated, the *mean point* will be the highest with matching sides on the bell-shaped curve.) The *median* point is the middle point with half the numbers on either side. The *mode* is the largest number at the top of the curve graph. It will be the most frequent result. If entering data to describe the range of a disease, no part of the data should be eliminated as it must remain a part of the graph. A good question might be *"what is the range of normal in this distribution?"*

Significantly, the bottom line is that a clinical study's *Abstract* is certainly not the whole story and the diligent representative will deeply reach into each Medical Study to learn the clinical aspects. Then, you will be ready to present a patient aspect of a clinical study and answer questions that providers may have.

"We should get out of an experience the wisdom that is in it, and stop there. Otherwise, he will be like the cat that sits on a hot stove lid. The Cate will never sit on a hot stove lid again, and that is good. But, It will never sit on a cold stove lid either" —Mark Twain

FACTORS DETERMINING STUDY DESIGN & IF RESULTS OF STUDY RELIABLE & VALID

Validity is all about whether or not the study results are statistically sound.

Reliability, another term mentioned relative to measurement, deals with the results of a study and how closely the results of the study could be reproduced by another group of researchers if they did the same study. This is absolutely necessary for the study to be valid.

So what **other factors** go into determining the design and whether the results are valid and reliable?

- **Patient population.**

  Eligibility, and importantly, which patients were excluded from the study. They were looking for clean data, not necessarily the range of patients that most physician offices and clinics see. Look to the sub-groups and numbers to make learn if they are of interest to your audience.

- **Clinical and Laboratory Evaluations**.

  The types of laboratory tests conducted in the study. If you plan to be viewed as a consultant by the customers you call on, and be able to enter into discussions with physicians relative to how this study can apply to them, referring to specific patient types and cases, it is important for you to know and understand the lab tests used in the study. Some of the lab tests may be available on a routine basis; others may be expensive and time-consuming. You may need to verify testing use and procedures to see if they are available in the community or *"only found in studies."*

- **Psychological Tests**---if these were used, they will be discussed here

- **Study Accrual**---

This is where the number of patients randomized (or entered the study) is shown in relation to the number of patients who completed the study._Pay close attention to which arms of the study had more dropouts and **WHY**. Placebo? Delivery system? High dose? Interesting to note. There may be a figure or chart that explains these numbers. Take time to see what the numbers might mean to the practitioner starting a patient on your product. Often, the reasons for discontinuance are given in this section.

- **Statistical Methods**--- The method of analysis of data will be outlined.

"There is no elevator to success---you have to take the stairs"
– Anonymous

KEY PHARMACOLOGY/PHARMACOKINETIC POINTS TO UNDERSTAND:

Half-Life, Area Under The Curve and P-Value

- **P-value**---when reading and analyzing medical studies you will encounter the phrase *"statistically significant"*. You will also encounter something called a *"P-Value"*. *"Customer Analytics for Dummies"* perhaps explains it best...

"In principle, a statistically significant result (usually a difference) is a result that is attributed to chance. More technically, it means that if the Null Hypothesis is true (which means there is no difference) there's a low probability of getting a result that is large or larger."

A small p-value (typically <0.05) indicates strong evidence against the null hypothesis so one rejects the null hypothesis which is a coin-toss likelihood. The "Null Hypothesis" defined: *"the hypothesis states that there is no significant difference between specified populations, any observed difference being do to sampling or experimental error."* Thus, small p-values are better in general. It is good to judge the p-value to see if it carries clinical relevance. Researchers determine where on the graph to start and stop measuring to show p-value. Biostatisticians have great fun developing these measures. Will the result predict clinical outcome?

- **Half-Life**

This term does not mean that the drug will be gone from the patient at the end of one additional half-life. Think of a bouncing ball. The first bounce comes up to ¾ of the distance dropped. The second bounce may rise to ½ the distance and when timed from the drop of the ball, gives the rate of elimination as well as when half of the drug remains in the body. Know that the ball will keep bouncing, shorter and shorter, and it can be quite a while before the ball is still.

Elimination rate is the result of either reactivation by the liver's hepatic chemistry, or renal function. Imagine graphing the bouncing ball with the goal of keeping the blood therapeutic level above the minimal effective amount. As the bounces drop to that level, another dose is given or ball is dropped.

That is why some drugs are Q.D., or once in 24-hours, or B.I.D., or once in 12-hours. More frequent dosing is very challenging to comply with and can raise compliance questions in study analysis

USING 'HALF LIFE' IN A PRESENTATION:

Understanding this aspect of pharmaceutical dosing will add believability beyond simply quoting your package insert's dosing guidelines:

Doctor, this drug has a loading dose that will get higher blood levels sooner to result in improved short term therapeutic responses! Why? Because 'Half Life' means that <u>half</u> the drug has been inactivated or excreted in that time interval. IMPORTANTLY, THE SECOND HALF LIFE DOES NOT MEAN THE DRUG IS COMPLETELY GONE FROM THE BODY! Dose interval is paired with the therapeutic concentration needed for efficacy. That therapeutic window is between too high at the upper level, and too low at the lower level in the blood or tissue. It is just like a bouncing ball that keeps bouncing, a little lower with each bounce. Following doses at regular intervals will continue to keep the blood levels in the desired therapeutic range for best results.

Compliance is a key part of the dosing, as you need to be aware that the more times a drug is taken in 24 hours, the lower the patient compliance will be. Pharmacologists measure hours between each dose and the delay of taking a dose is regarded as a dosing error in the hospital.

Thus, it is good to have drugs that are "1 Q.D. = 1 in 24 hours" as that dosing has the highest patient compliance. "1 B.I.D. = 1 every 12 hours" also has high compliance. Since your product is one of those two intervals, compliance will be best and the results more likely and predictable. Doctor, you

know that "1 T.I.D. = every 8 hours" or "1 Q.I.D. = every 6 hours" will have much lower compliance.
https://www.ncbi.nlm.nih.gov/pmc/articles/PMC4283966/

- Area Under The Curve

  A pharmacokinetic term that understands that drug concentrations may vary with the kind of drug administered to a patient. Drug concentration peaks and the highest after administration, then drops off as metabolism or excretion reduce the drug to the trough before the next dose.

  The term refers to all the area that is *"drug"* and is under the line from administration to trough and shows how likely there will be therapeuticconcentration in a patient for a measured amount of time.

  A drug with a smaller peak, but faster elimination, will have a smaller Area Under The Curve (AUC).

"Originality is unexplored territory. You get there by canoe, you can't take a taxi" —Alan Alda

BIAS

1. Bias In Clinical Studies…If The Goal Is Clinical Relevance, How Can Study Bias Cloud Significance?

2. How To Spot Bias In All The Right Places

BIAS IN CLINICAL STUDIES

The word "bias" in clinical studies is vastly different from the bias used in the public press. Additionally, there are two terms that must be understood before we go to to the rest of the subject.

They are ***"Incidence"*** and ***"Prevalence"*** They are <u>not</u> interchangeable. <u>Prevalence</u> is the number of cases in the general total population. *Incidence* gives the number, for example, of cases from the above *Prevalence* that are seen by a specific specialty. Specialists see referred patients from general practitioners and thus see a higher percentage of that specific type of case. Their impression of the number of cases will be higher due to the *incidence* in their practices. The difference in these terms is something to pay attention to when reading clinical studies. If you are preparing a presentation to a specific specialty group, you need to focus upon any studies from that specialty as their *incidence* will be higher.

We strongly believe that your goal is to identify one or two patient types who would most benefit from a trial with your therapy. Here there are many challenging aspects in design and interpretation that may alter the value of a clinical study. These patient types can be determined only by a lot of time spent with clinical studies and also discussions with insightful clinicians.

This section on BIAS will help you develop an ability to look critically and objectively at clinical studies. Combining this relatively large amount of information with deep knowledge of pharmacokinetics of your product as well as your competition will help you towards your goal.

Remember that clinicians already are using the products that they have found to be most often effective and they have memorized all aspects of their dosing so that they can confidently respond to DX-RX questions at any time of the day or night. You are seeking a way to help them know why to remember an additional clinical therapeutic point.

It is the goal of medical clinical studies to establish what works best with the majority of patients, focusing upon patient outcome.

When evaluating clinical studies, there are a number of aspects that can raise questions about how the results were obtained. Starting with the least valuable data would be the people doing TV and internet advertising, who state that their approach yielded the desired favorable result on this single example, implying that other people should try whatever it was.

At best, these are referred to as anecdotes, since they involve only one approach and usually very few people and no negative outcomes. There is no clinical significance to these results, and anecdotes are of minimal interest.

The basic starting point:

There are *"gold standard"* designs of clinical studies such as--- double blind, placebo control, and randomizing. Institutions have IRBs, or Investigational Review Boards, that oversee what data can be collected about their patients. Well designed and implemental studies return their value over time though some clinicians doubt studies not done more recently. Clinical studies form the basis to what is referred to as *"evidence-based medicine"*

One cannot simply look at a clinical study and determine if bias was present at any point so that a 'yes' or 'no' is easily determined. Also, these determinations are usually partial and incremental.

How To Spot Bias

Seeking BIAS requires an insightful mindset, combined with cynicism, doubt and skepticism. We are daily lulled into acceptance by TV ads that show single highly successful comparisons of *"before and after"* products are used.

One final point here, and a key one…by knowing how to analyze the "*Material & Methods*" section of a paper, you learn how to analyze an article and make your own decision on whether or not, you the reader, can believe the results and understand if they are relevant and timely. These are the best anecdotes, and their intent is to convince viewers that their results will always be good as the single example shown.

With clinical studies, much more depth is needed. There are guidelines to follow in the design of these studies though those are not always followed and the guidelines are fairly recently developed.

We acknowledge that there are pages of many different aspects to BIAS in medical studies---we are going to focus on only a few of more blatant ones that might be questioned by an astute reader. The basic goal of studies is to improve the outcome of a certain group of patients, while saving treatment dollars.

With the general example of a double-blinded study with 2-arms (treatment and placebo)----

1. The planned study is submitted to the institution's IRB or Investigational Review Board since no data can be collected from their patients without their approval.

2. The study will have a goal,

3. And have methods to evaluate patients to see efficacy in the study towards that goal

4. Hopefully, that goal will be valuable and assist clinicians in making the best choices for treatment

5. Hidden BIAS can occur if a different aspect of the outcome is not considered or anticipated in the study---

6. Question if the patients studied could have another cause for their disease that is not evaluated

7. The depth of control of the "double-blind" aspect is important as ideally none of the participants know the code and thus cannot control when each patient is placed

When the authors select the points of measure for their study, they may exclude "outliers" that fall outside the main body of patient responses. A number of patients will be "lost to follow up" and cannot be tracked. Sometime medical issues, adverse effects, or even death are reasons for their data not being available. Incomplete data is a BIAS. These patients should be discussed in some detail within the paper as their absence may affect the overall study goal.

The investigators choose the parameters used to create their 'p' value, so that is why we pay attention to the following:

1. Patients lost to the study

2. Exclusions

3. Other reasons for not including the original number of patients in the study

The number of patients is important. This is referred to as the 'n' or number.

Generally, larger numbers are more expensive while providing better accuracy. If the disease studied is rare, there will not be a very large number studied. Smaller numbers of rare diseases may indicate a need for larger studies involving many research hospitals. Internal medicine specialists tend to remember these small studies and focus upon them to a greater degree than others who will reward small numbers of events as mere anecdotal mentions.

Definitions of '*Anecdote*'

a. Not necessarily true or reliable, because based on personal accounts rather than facts or research

b. Based on or consisting of reports or observations of usually unscientific observers

c. Anecdotal information is not based on facts or careful study

d. Based on reports or things someone saw rather than on proven facts

Sometimes *retrospective studies* are undertaken to increase the number of patients analyzed. These studies go back to all the papers published on that patient aspect. They are exhaustive and require a lot of work to compile. Due to the many different sites and dates, there will be minimal consistency in the kinds of tests and evaluations run as each study was designed by different researchers. The kinds of patients dropped from the studies will be different and those lost to follow-up will yield questions.

Ask yourself, "*what patients were not included at "trial end?*". Also, "*are unfavorable results a part of the focus?*" Some side effects occur may not occur until sometime after the active portion of a trial. Were there follow-up examinations to measure delayed side effects? In what detail were adverse events included? If none, that would indicate **BIAS.**

A major BIAS error is to compare the retrospective studies on an *"even playing field"*, pretending that all their outcomes are equivalent and contribute to a single conclusion. At times the reference was not a major end point for some of the studies, it was just mentioned in some of the laboratory studies (even a *'standard lab test'* will yield different results at different research hospitals). Over time, lab tests most valued will change as newer ones are devised and replace old ones. Constructing sub-groups of patients and then analyzing their separate 'p' values can produce results that need deeper analysis.

BIAS can result from the inclusion of different groups of patients. The pharmacological therapy response is not straight line between children and the elderly, it rises and falls through life so that the elderly should be a separate analytical group in many studies.

They have decreased body mass, lower metabolism and reduced end-organ function. Major medical centers have patients with thicker charts as they have been referred due to their challenges and they may be more difficult to evaluate along with other patients with only one or a few medical challenges. The daily dosing of treatments can also be a BIAS factor, as compliance decreases as the number of times a product is dosed increases. To compare 1 Q.24-hour's efficacy with 1 Q. 6-hours can yield weakened comparisons.

Another BIAS error is to extract one or a small handful of studies from the many cited, to make a point towards a single conclusion.

The expense of larger studies must be paid. The funding source needs to be mentioned along with other support for the study. This includes the researchers themselves who may be paid speakers or own stock in the company with the product being evaluated. Recently, these have been listed within the studies and the reader needs to make note of those relationships.

Reproducible results are a cornerstone of scientific research. An example of this challenge occurred in the evaluation of vaccine side effects, as the findings were not reproducible.

Now you have some insightful reasons to go beyond a study's abstract, to delve into the methods used to find those results. You will be able to see if treatment changes are warranted, and your time will be well spent.

THE BRIEFING GUIDE ©

We developed the **"Briefing Guide"**© (see end of manual) to assist you in asking pertinent and important questions about the medical journal article you are reviewing. The Guide is good in helping you keep a record of important medical studies you have reviewed. If you need to refer back on a study, the *"Guide"* makes it easy for you to do so.

TERMS YOU NEED TO KNOW...

Crossover design. The patients in the original arms of the study are all simultaneously given the other therapy, or treatment method. In this way, patient variability is much reduced as a factor.

Crossover. Alternates patients in a study.

Double-Blinded Trial. Neither investigator nor patient is aware if placebo or active product is used for any patient participating in study.

Experimental design. The structure of the study, with the goal of producing a measurable effect from the clinical effort.

Inter-patient variability. Certainly all patients are not identical, and these differences need to be considered to see if study results might have been influenced.

Open-label. Everyone knows what each patient is being given. It is felt that the study outcome will be great enough that blinding or use of placebos is either not necessary, or it is not possible.

Placebo. A critical concept. This is a preparation that appears just like the real therapeutic product, although there is nothing inside that is therapeutically active. Typically called a 'sugar pill'. The difference between this "zero" therapy and the active one is measured during studies.

Placebo-controlled. The use of two look-alike preparations in a clinical study. One is the active product, and the other is an inactive preparation that will be randomly be given to study patients. The results of the active product is compared to those of the placebo at the end of the study once the 'codes' are broken and studied. In this way, the efficacy of the active treatment can be measured against a known, controlled patient population.

Population. During a study, all of the patients enrolled on all arms of the study are the Population. There are also Populations in each arm of the study, and it is the goal of the study that each arm match so that the results can be seen more clearly.

Prospective. Looking forward in time. More studies are requested.

p-Value. A p-value of less than 5% (0.5) is statistically significant or unlikely due to chance. The break points are decided by the authors.

Randomization. A method of assigning patients to different treatments, or arms, of a study. This can be done in a random manner so that neither the patients nor the physicians know what is being given.

Retrospective. Looking backward in time, referring to many prior studies.

RESULTS

This section is worth a lot of study and presents information on what happened when the study was conducted. This is where those p-values are reported. Make absolutely sure you understand all of the terminology used. Don't be afraid to ask someone about a word or phrase so that you can better get a grasp on what is being said. Concomitant illnesses and medications might be mentioned here. Would they influence outcome?

Charts, figures, diagrams and tables are presented in the results section. Study these carefully paying particular attention to things that are exceptions or that stand out. It is interesting to read the list of things that were NOT statistically significant to the study – think about WHY and if that pertains to every day practice or not. Sometimes these were not significant because the drug did not work that well. What patients benefited the most? Least? It is important for you to know both.

From a presenter's perspective, these charts, diagrams and tables can really support and illustrate your point, just as they do in the paper. Most of the sales literature used by pharmaceutical representatives contains charts showing favorable study results. They are a lot stronger when put in the context of the original study.

Nota Bene

The point to be made here is presenting a chart or a diagram to an audience without knowing the design of the study and how the results were obtained is not a consultative approach. Would it not be a lot smarter to know how the study was designed, the patient population, tests conducted, etc in case your audience asks you a question when you present a chart or diagram showing results of a study? Results given out of context really supply little value to you or your customer.

DISCUSSION SECTION

Information presented in this section can run the gamut from comments comparing this paper with past papers to comments about the results of the study. From your perspective, because this section is usually the most interesting section of a paper, use it to help build your presentation.

You can get a lot of good quotes from the Discussion section of an article to use in a presentation. These are often wonderful insights or thought starters that can get a real conversation going with your physician. Remember to keep to your point and guide the conversation. Many an attention span has been lost by going into academic *"discussions"* that are unlikely to improve any office patient outcomes.

Because there is rarely a final, all-questions-answered study, as patients and their infections change over time, many times in the Discussion Section of a paper you will see comments by the authors may suggest, *"Further studies may be needed"*. These should be read in context, and completely. They do NOT invalidate the findings, but are guide posts for future work the authors feel is needed.

Nota Bene

You can get a lot of good quotes from the Discussion section of an article to use in a sales presentation. These are often wonderful openings or thought starters that can get a real conversation going with your audience.

THE REFERENCES

The reference section of an article is also called the <u>bibliography sectio</u>n. Here the authors disclose the sources for the information that they are using, if it is not part of the study. This is the original source of the information. At times, studies cited in the references will be highly important to the findings.

From a presenter's perspective, this section of the paper gives a pretty good idea of how well the authors <u>researched the past literature,</u> and an idea of the scope. Secondly, the reference section provides an excellent opportunity to see what articles you have read and haven't read.

Note the authors the papers used as references. The more cross-referencing in a paper, the more it is demonstrating a preponderance of the evidence, and the more likely the paper will make an impact on how your treatment is used. This is what is meant by _"evidence-based medicine"_ and is highly important to improving specific patient outcomes or quality of life.

Check the years noted for the early references on the subject. These early articles usually describe the disease and what is known about the disease. These are called epidemiological studies because they describe the disease and its prevalence, without studying treatment. Check the references listed for anecdotal papers. These studies are called _"anecdotal papers"_ as they are not controlled studies. Papers like this do provide insight into treatment possibilities, but are not part of evidence-based medicine.

If you find a reference that looks important and relevant to the point you are trying to make, go look it up. Knowing the background will give you more confidence.

"If you do your lessons every night, you never have to worry about a test" — U.J. Hecker

SUMMARY: QUICK INSIGHTS...
HOW TO APPROACH A CLINICAL STUDY

Analyzing Medical Studies

These comments should apply to clinical studies in general. Collecting patient data requires Investigational Review Board approval, and must be very well recorded. Studies are very expensive!

Authors

- Where was the study done?

- Was there more than one study site? (if more than one, we will be watchful to see how carefully each site has aligned their testing, randomization and therapy)

- Did the authors have any financial interest in the study outcome?

- Are their paid speakers presenting the study to various medical groups?

Abstract

Often times readers do not have time to go beyond this overview. It can yield some insight into questions about study organization, analysis and reporting. Often a date of journal submission is listed. If there is a significant pause in time between that date and the date of the journal publication, ask yourself why?

What Was Study Designed To Analyze

- Is the data going to be helpful to improve selected patient outcome with new insight?

- In other words, are the results valuable for your patient outcomes?

- How many patients were entered?

- How many patients completed the study?

INTRODUCTION

The introduction is an overview. Medical Center patients are more complex since they have been referred from the community, and thus patient analysis may show different aspects of incidence and prevalence from your community practice patients.

The bottom line is to answer the question, *"how might this study change the way my patients are tested and treated?"*

Limitations…ask what limitations were placed upon the study patients testing and treatment that might not apply to the patients you see and treat. Often medical center tests are not covered by community patient insurance plans.

Material & Methods

These allow the authors to determine cutoff points and acceptable ranges of results that will vary from those available to the community practices, and also allow the authors to choose *"windows of analysis"* for p-values.

Results

The population characteristics are worth looking into. Particularly check to see starting population size versus those completing the study.

- Why did those patients not stay with the study?

- Were the patients eliminated by the authors?

- If so, where is the analysis of those patients? They may have had characteristics that would have changed the p-value, or they may have had other aspects found during work-up that necessitated their removal. All of these should be noted in the study to enhance credibility

Adverse Effects?

There may have been reasons for discontinuing a small group of patients, and you want to know what those findings were

Discussion

Look for insights here that may provide reasons to change patient testing or treatment if they are strong enough.

Patient Follow-Up

How much effort was expended in contacting those patients who did not report for their clinical visits? This is an area of focus upon, and insight gained from your patient population may help you understand some of these aspects.

Conclusion

This is a very good place to visit---it usually asks for further studies, of course. Aside from that constant, this section should place the study findings into perspective about how these authors regard the placement and value of their results.

Ask, *"does this apply to my patients, or is there a patient I know of who could benefit from these insights"?*

Then, The References

Read through them to see what other studies the authors looked at, what the publication dates are and ask if there are perhaps a couple of them you want to request and study.

"The lion and the tiger may be more powerful, but the wolf does not perform in the circus" --Anonymous

MAKING THE CLINICAL STUDY RELEVANT: FITTING IT INTO YOUR AUDIENCE'S THOUGHT PROCESSES

Your primary goal is to fit your presentation and the use of a reprint into a treater's established thought-sequence. So, what is that?

When a patient diagnosis is made (DX), the next thought is of therapeutic options (RX). A lot goes into that diagnosis. That is the art and science of medicine.

As a treater progresses through their residency, they continue a sequence of rotations through different specialties or clinics, all designed to teach the type of patient and what to *"expect"*. Clinicians begin to mentally sort through the tremendous varieties of patient conditions and begin to learn how to test and diagnose. A major part of their study is devoted to going from signs and symptoms to the reasons for the best tests to conduct. Their memories are focused on identifying key clinical signs and symptoms, then choosing tests that will narrow the variety of possible diagnoses, then treating.

Often this sequence is described as going from a differential diagnosis, using carefully chosen tests, to a presumptive diagnosis, and then selecting a treatment therapy.

This continues throughout a medical career, whether in discussions with colleagues or at meetings, there is a *"sequence"* of presenting the information

- Patient Background: Gender, ethnicity, age, weight

- Chief patient complaint(s)

- Laboratory workup and results

- Presumptive diagnosis with possible additional tests

- Summary diagnosis and course of treatment

For a particular patient in an office, this works like a series of *"toggle switches"* like this:

- Adult-----------------click

- Female---------------click

- Normal BP-----------click

- Pain------------------click

- Diabetes-------------click

- Took product 'A' for 6-months---click

- Kidneys declining in function-----click

Mental note: Product 'B' might be a better choice – it is not excreted by the kidneys!

The value of a specific patient description along with charts and diagrams

The challenge is to understand this *'sequence'* of how clinicians are trained to think and make decisions so an advantage can be identified that can be inserted into one of the *'toggles'*. Identifying a specific competitive advantage your therapy has in one of the *"toggle switches"* might be an evaluation of kidney function. Treatment goal is to insert a therapeutic advantage that relates to a specific patient type – in the example above, the subtype might be a diabetic with declining renal function.

Read the study. Break it down to understand it. Make it relevant to the clinician's practice you are presenting the study to. The goal is to improve patient outcome. We can't stress this enough.

We discuss in-depth *"patient-type centered"*© selling in our book **"How To Sell Pharmaceuticals & Medical Devices When You Are Really Not Sure How"** available from Sheeley Consulting Group, LLC. The book teaches what no other sales book on the market does, and that is, how physicians are trained to think and make drug selection decisions. For if you know this, you know how to present a product that makes sense to the physician.

SUMMARY:

The key to learning how to read, understand and interpret the medical literature lies in first knowing the importance of the "Materials and Methods" section of an article and in knowing what to look for in an article, e.g., study design and results.

It takes a lot of time and effort to learn how to understand and interpret the medical literature. But, the more one reads, the better one gets at really knowing how to dissect a paper and how to use key results from a paper. Plan to help a specific patient type by focusing the study data into proper patient perspectives in sales presentations.

Knowing how to read and understand the medical literature is the road less traveled in pharmaceutical sales, but the effort separates the outstanding from the average.

The insights you have gained in the analysis and understanding of Clinical Studies are vital to apply to each Medical Study that you read. You will enjoy the deeper insights learned from studies in the future.

Those skills will give you academic confidence and earn you respect when you discuss the finer points with your prescribers as well.

"It is what you learn after you know it all that really counts" – John Wooden

HOW TO FOCUS PATIENT-SPECIFIC ATTENTION ON YOUR POINT, OR,

THE NEXT STEP TO PREPARE A PRESENTATION:

L earn and memorize the key therapeutic points within your product's package insert.

If there is either a main competitor or class of competitors, examine their clinical studies with the skills you have just learned. Mentally compare them with your clinical study. You might even prepare a two column chart for your own study. Of course, this would never be used in the field. Learn the package inserts of others in your marketplace. They are excellent sources for your preparatory comparisons.

Now, with those four sources of insight (two package inserts and two Clinical studies), look at subset advantages your therapy may have, as well as subsets of shortcomings your competition may have in comparison with yours. Examples = Hepatic elimination/inactivation? Renal elimination?

Begin to create what will be an introductory outline, based upon how residents present chart reviews to attendings and staff members. **Your goal is to use a similar pathway of discussion, because you will be creating a mental picture of a patient sitting on their examining table during an examination.** Use their abbreviations – HR for heart rate, and so forth. They use abbreviation codes to save everyone time. Note the gender, weight, age, renal function, other concurrent maladies, and current prescriptions. The latter choices will increasingly focus upon your specific patient, giving almost everything that is necessary. You will soon have a short list that points in a pretty focused direction. *Your insights will be valuable to help focus this sequence.* Then, you will likely want to mention a lab test result that will help bring the treater's mind into the treatment room and their mental differential diagnosis will kick in with a very short list of possibilities. Then, you might mention the most common diagnosis and therapy (DX/RX).

Next comes your point to remember: this patient was treated with (generic name or category of therapy), and because of their renal function and the extended half-life of the one used, along with a reported interaction with one of their maintenance drugs (_____) a situation exists to try (your treatment) for the first time. "Does that sound reasonable? How will you remember this until that infrequent patient is sitting in your exam room? Also, since this will be a first use for you, the Rx is written this way, with the "1 Q.D," or, "apply Q.D." and mention that it is most effectively at bedtime. The most common side effect is _____, and only Q_____ interacts by decreasing efficacy."

The reason for this last important comment about interactions and side effects is because that first use will be closely watched for any untoward patient responses. Sometimes it is wise to allude to the thought that might say, *"You will likely be trying (my product name) on some fairly challenging patients and the chances of side effects and so forth may be a bit higher in your first patients than the later ones."* Also, this sequence has provided your clinician with a reason to refuse a general therapeutic substitution by managed care, as it is a rare case when that usual first choice would be much less desirable.

It may be days or even weeks until your clinician has a chance to try your product, so on a next visit you may wish to reinforce the diagnostic spot seeking that new use, and perhaps mention something else helpful, such as coverage in managed care. Providers don't enjoy pharmacy call-backs requesting a change in prescription.

TERMS YOU NEED TO KNOW

Cohort Study: This is a group of patients within a study. This subset may have been found to have different results from the main body of the study. Often, these cohorts lack sufficient members to yield statistical validity.

Concordance: Agreement.

Crossover design: The patients in the original arms of the study are all simultaneously given the other therapy, or treatment method. In this way, patient variability is much reduced as a factor.

Crossover: To alternate patients in a study.

Double-Blinded Trial: Neither investigator nor patient is aware if placebo or active drug being used for any patient participating in study.

Experimental design: The structure of the study, with the goal of producing a measurable effect from the clinical effort while minimizing any chance of design bias.

False negatives: Test result that is reported as negative, when the actual patient is positive. This can occur along with the following:

False positives: When a test result is positive, when the actual existence is negative. False negatives and false positives are examples of how tests are not necessarily 100% accurate. As those reasons become better understood, and the percentage of their existence is more accurately known, a test may be known as, for example, 95% accurate. In those outlying situations where the physician wants to be certain of the test result, there is another, or different test that can confirm or deny the initial result.

Grand Rounds: Meetings attended by residents, fellows, attendings and community physicians to review and discuss patient-types via cases and journal articles.

Inference: A generalization, or opinion based upon a best guess.

Informed consent: This is a form that patients sign whenever a medical procedure is to be performed on them. In the case of a clinical study, the form may describe the possible untoward effects, and state that the outcome cannot be guaranteed or known, due to the use of, for example, placebo, products or preparations that are approved only for trial on selected patients. Studies with informed consent are the major way new products come to market.

Inter-patient variability: The recognition that all patients are not identical, and how these differences need to be considered to see if study results might have been influenced.

Investigational Review Board (IRB): This board exists in most large hospitals and medical centers and assures that patient confidentiality and ethics are followed in the design and methodology of a study. The purpose of the Board is to review any proposed collection of data from the patient population that is seen there. The result is that patient confidentiality is protected and the collection of any data is only through protocols that have been read and approved by the IRB.

Mean: Average.

Median. The middle, or most representative part of the study results.

Meta-analysis: An analysis that combines results from more than one study. These results may be intellectually interesting, but they do not carry the weight of a single study. Also called Retrospective studies. The reason is that all of the controls and tests in one test are almost never carried out by another study, so the results are understood to not be universal. Often used to add together many studies so that larger numbers of patients with similar diagnoses can be compared.

Observational bias: If the clinician or observer knows which patients are assigned to each arm of the study, they may be looking for specific outcomes in a prejudiced way.

Open-label: Everyone knows what drug each patient is being given. It is felt that the study outcome will be great enough that blinding or use of placebos is either not necessary, or it is not possible.

Parameters: The guidelines and 'rules' of the study.

Peer-reviewed: The paper, study or presentation has been read and examined by other experts in that particular field and found to be solid in terms of the science and importance to advancing the practice of medicine. It is the "thumbs up" review of credibility. Many key medical journals use this approach before publishing.

Placebo: A critical concept. This is a preparation that appears just like the real therapeutic dose, although there is nothing inside that is therapeutically active. Typically called a 'sugar pill'. The difference between this "zero" therapy and the active one is measured during studies.

Placebo-controlled: The use of two look-alike preparations in a clinical study. An inactive 'drug' (the placebo) is given to certain patients in the study and the active drug is given to others. The results of the active drugs are compared to those of the placebo at the end of the study once the 'codes' are broken and studied. In this way, the efficacy of the active drug can be measured against a known, controlled patient population.

Population: During a study, all of the patients enrolled on all arms of the study are the Population. There are also Populations in each arm of the study, and it is the goal of studies that each arm matches so that the results can be seen more clearly.

Powering a study: A statistical term that understands how many patients must be seen to measure a certain response. Some studied questions may take in excess of 20,000 patients to get enough actual responses of an infrequent diagnosis so that a result can be published that is statistically significant.

Prospective: Looking forward in time.

Random allocation: Assigning subjects in a study to keep it non-biased.

Randomization: A method of assigning patient to different treatments, or arms, of a study. This can be done in a random manner so that neither the patients nor the physicians know what is being given.

Retrospective: Looking backward in time, at a number of previously published studies. It is unlikely that all aspects of previous studies and designs are duplicated.

Standard Deviation: A statistically accepted variable.

Statistically significant: When the study is analyzed by a statistical method, a "*p*-" value is assigned, and the smaller that the "*p*-" value is, the more significant, or pronounced, the results. There are a number of biostatistical kinds of data analysis.

Stratified randomization: Possible break points assigned to make certain that the severity of symptoms is dealt with so that each level of patient is entered into therapy that is aligned with their needs.

Validity: In this context, validity is expressed as a statistical number. The greater the difference between, for example, placebo and drug study, the more valid the test results.

Washout period: A time interval that comes before actual trial drugs and placebos are administered or between arms if there is crossover. During this time, patients who were on certain other medications are given time for the effects of both of those drugs and their metabolites to leave the patient's bodies. The result is that effects measured during the study can be more accurately assigned to the study results.

Washout Period: Often, patients will be admitted to a study that are already on a therapy for the indication being studied. They will wait, with no drug therapy, while the drug and its metabolites leave their bodies. That is the washout period, and then the patients can be assigned to treatment per the study design.

"The art of being wise is the ability to know what to over look" --William James

SELF- STUDY

WHAT TO READ IN THE TIME YOU HAVE

There are too many articles with many good intentions to read all that is published. The day never arrives when you have the time to read *'nice to know'* articles. Be selective in your reading and concentrate your reading efforts and time on the following:

- Studies and case reports involving your drug and your competitor's product.

- Major peer-reviewed journals.

- Journal articles reviewing new laboratory tests involving your product.

- Journal articles dealing with disease state involving your product.

- Articles that review new approaches. (e.g., The Medical Letter).

WHERE TO GO TO FIND JOURNAL ARTICLES OF VALUE TO YOUR SUCCESS

First, go to your product's package insert (P.I.). Your P.I. is an underutilized key reference that has been thoroughly approved. Examples of areas that are important: half-life, active metabolites, and route of excretion.

Next, get a copy of your past literature or the core visual aid. You will see a place where there are *'references'*. There will not be many references listed, and you may need to go to the medical library or Medline and obtain a copy of each of these papers from the journals they were published in. Study these to learn vocabulary and study aspects.

OTHER TYPES OF ARTICLES OR PUBLICATIONS YOU MAY ENCOUNTER

Editorials and Letters to the Editor

Editorials provide opinions and it is important to learn what other experts found important in the article. Letters raise questions. Questions are good, but lit is important to remember that letters are not peer-reviewed. Like any letter, they are an opinion.

There is no peer review.

When confronted with a Letter or Editorial that speaks unfavorably about your therapy, take the high road. Don't get confrontational. You do not know if your audience agrees or not.

Case Reports

Case reports have appeared in the medical literature for many years. These show how guidelines, studies, and "*best practice*" are put into a reality check with real patients. Pay particular attention to how the case is broken down and presented to the reader. That is the constant sequence a physician uses when working with patients.

You will want to be aware of and read case reports reviewing specific patient types. A good case report will be referenced and show WHY a physician made the decisions she/he did.

Studies on Small Numbers of Patients

There is another part of medical publications that is particularly interesting to specialists. Studies on small groups of patients, say 1 to 20-patients, are often regarded as anecdotal. That does not mean they are invalid, only that they do not have the statistical power that the larger studies do. They often form the basis for a larger, more significant study.

White Paper. A scientific paper published for medical decision-making and serving as an insight or background. These can be authoritative and advocate a position or approach to understand a therapy or to present an aspect of treatment. Their use needs corporate approval.

JOURNAL ARTICLES IN ACTION: LEARN HOW PHYSICIANS PUT PAPER TO PRACTICE

Journal Clubs

Journal club meetings are a great place to see first-hand how a journal article is dissected and discussed by physicians. Journal clubs take place within hospital departments, for example infectious disease, anesthesia, etc. Ask the Chief Resident if you can attend to listen and learn. Get the schedule and see what articles will be reviewed and discussed and who is assigned to lead the discussion. Attend the meeting.

<u>What to look for</u>:

- How the presenter provides an '<u>*overview*</u>' of the paper under discussion.

- How study <u>design</u> is discussed.

- The types of questions asked, and how the 'presenter' answered the questions. Did the 'presenter' discuss:

  - study design?

  - Number of patients enrolled?

  - Side effects?

  - Results?

- What did the '*presenter*' review in the '*results*' section?

- Comments the '*presenter*' made about the '*discussion*' section?

Grand Rounds/Specialty Conferences

A great place to see how cases are discussed and how medical journal articles are broken-down and discussed. The presenter shows slides of the key reprints discussed in the case and it is to your advantage to see how a reprint is broken down and shown on a slide. These programs are held routinely in teaching medical centers, and are usually open to sales representatives. Papers discussed at grand rounds conferences are usually of interest to physicians in private practice and offer an easy entry into getting a doctor's attention.

M&M (Morbidity & Mortality) conferences

M&M conferences are the heart of learning for physicians. A review of the assessment, treatment and outcomes for patients who did not have a good outcome (significant morbidity or mortality) are presented. Any treaters who were involved with the patient at any level are present and will justify their approaches. The entire staff discusses ways to improve their approach to that specific patient type to ensure that any future patients, who are similar, will be treated differently to improve outcomes.

National Meetings, poster sessions

National meetings are specialty focused, and members who have studies under way are chosen to present their significant new studies or insights. There are often rooms of Poster Sessions where posters are on easels, with an author present, and their materials and methods are often included.

USING MEDICAL JOURNAL STUDIES ("REPRINTS")
TO GAIN MARKET SHARE---ADVANCED COURSE

This approach assumes that you are already capable of reading and understanding a clinical study, also called a reprint.

You will need to access a medical library. These are found in big hospitals and medical centers. Ask a research librarian how the library is set up, and how to use the computer terminals if they have them.

Next, you will need to know the competitive products' generic names. *Visit with a clinical nurse* in the section where your drug would have use. Ask them what their challenges are, and what is important to them about how their patients progress clinically. Take notes! Prepare to answer those concerns with your study and preparation, for *specific patient types*.

Let's start with your product

First, go to your package insert (called the "P.I."). It is assumed that you have learned it, and know where to find answers that may come up. Your P.I. can become a key reference.

Examples: Half Life? Active Metabolites? Route of Excretion?

Next, get a piece of your detailing sales literature, or your core visual aid. You will see a place where there are "References". There will not be many, and you need to go to the medical library and photo-copy each of these papers from the journals they were published in. If you can get a piece of literature from your competition, you will need to get copies of their referenced studies, as well. *You are looking for patient types where your product has a clear patient outcome advantage.* Don't try to to go for all patients at once.

Now, your preparation started

Let's use an example of a paper published in JAMA, the weekly journal of the American Medical Association. We are going to "*take it apart*" to see what's there, and how it can help us. Make marks! This is a study copy. You have the date of the issue.

Look at the lower left part of the front page---sometimes you can see when a paper was submitted to the journal. If it had a prolonged wait, there were questions that had to be answered before being published. Also, this is where the funding came from. Neutral sources are more highly regarded than pharmaceutically supported studies.

In the abstract under the title of the paper, there are around 9-sections. This is where doctors spend their reading time.

Content gives the overview for where the paper is designed to fit

Objective gives what they wanted to do

Design is important;_double-blinded, randomized, placebo-controlled trials are very good. The researchers did not know what they were giving each patient, and they noted progress by charting changes after patient visits.

Setting can be interesting. Multiple sites are more likely to eliminate the chance that a single institution had a procedure that was unusual. On the other hand, it is harder to control variable when the study was done at many sites.

Participants tells how many patients they initially entered into the study.

Intervention tells how the drugs were administered, whether there was a washout or not, and so forth. The notation (n=976 means how many patients in that part of the study). When asked, "*What is the 'N' number?*" This is what they want to know---the total number of patients entered.

Main Outcome Measures are the things that the study found that were changes from a baseline, that were measured during the study.

Results are important, because this section is one that your providers read, and it will be interesting to see what the good and challenged parts of the results were.

In this section, they will use "p-values" shown as an example as "P=0.5" (which is NOT good enough, it takes a smaller number). The more zeros there are after the decimal, the better, because the tiniest number here is the most significant. Look for specific patient types you can discuss. (Examples: reduced renal function? Elderly? Elevated liver enzymes?)

Conclusions is the section that summarizes the paper to show what the authors think is the key overall finding. Your focus may not be in that direction, and you may be looking at other aspects of the study.

A Section That Is Not Titled that gives an overview for why the study was set up, and what they wanted to answer. This is the first time you will see little numbers, or superscripts, at the end of sentences. (example 12.16). These numbers relate to other clinical studies listed in the references section at the end of the paper. As you study the clinical study, if a statement is made that relates to the competitive situation in your hands, you will want to make a checkmark by that study in the References section.

Methods Study Design

This presents the design, and will discuss things such as *screening, washout, placebo period, titration period, and possibly a maintenance period.* You may note that some of the doses in the design are either above or below the ones that are approved for your presentation. When you get to the competitive studies, you will want to see what their studies dose levels were, as well.

Patient Population

Eligibility, and importantly, *which patients were excluded from the study.* They were looking for clean data, and necessarily using the range of patients that most offices and clinics see. Notice their randomized break points for the patients. You will need to learn the average lab values to see how these apply to patients in your clinics. This will give you a good background for discussions with physicians, because you will know their test data and language.

Clinical and Laboratory Evaluations

You may need to talk with a physician or nurse to see if the tests used and intervals set up are ones that have practical use in their practice. Compliance is at once both easy to measure and challenging to assure.

Psychological tests

If these were used, they will be discussed here

Study Accrual

This is where the number of patients randomized, (or who entered the study) are shown in relation to the number of patients who *completed* the study. Pay attention to which arms had more dropout. Placebo? Low dose? High dose? Interesting to note. There may be a figure, or chart that explains these number. Take some time to see what the numbers might mean to a practitioner starting a patient on your drug. Often, the reasons for discontinuance are given here.

Statistical Methods

From your standpoint, did they use means, or averages? What were the ranges? Ages? How are the studied patients different from the ones in your clinics?

Results

This section is worth a lot of study. Make sure you understand all of the terminology used. Do not be afraid to ask someone about a word or phrase so that you can better get a grasp on what is being said. Concomitant illnesses and medications might be mentioned here. Would they influence outcome? What percent of patients were titrated to the highest dose?

Note: This is where they discuss these p-values they discovered. It is interesting to read the list of things that were NOT statistically significant. Sometimes these were not significant because there were not enough patients in the study. Other times, it is because the drug didn't work that well. What patient types benefited the most? Least? Know both.

Charts, Figures and Tables

Study these carefully, noting things that are exceptions, or that stand out.

Comment

Here the authors of the study will make key statements and they will often be supported by a cite to a reference study listed at the end. If the comment pertains to your problem, make a checkmark by that clinical study under References.

One paper reviewed. Now, do the same with the rest of yours, checking reference papers you'll need in each one.

Action:

Now go back thru the library stacks and make copies of all the papers you checked.

If you have a piece of literature from your competition, you can now do the same sequence with their clinical studies, getting copies and studying sections discussed above.

If you do not have any references for you competition, you will want to go to the reference or research librarian, and ask for help doing a search on the indication and generic name of the product. (You can run one on your drug, as well, while you are at the terminal).

What you will learn is that the database can be huge for some products. Limit the search by selecting "human", "adult", "English language", and then ask for a *250-word truncated abstract search.* This will give you a brief description of each paper. As soon as it's entered, you will see how many studies they have found. If it is a small number of pages, have them print the list, so you can see what you have. Ask the librarian's help to indicate key journals so that you won't be wasting time with less impressive journals.

As a side note, there is another part of medical publications that is particularly interesting to specialists. Studies on small groups of patients, say from 1 to 20 patients are often regarded as *anecdotal.* That does not mean they are invalid, only that they do not have the statistical power that the larger studies do. If there are interesting references in this search list that involve only a few patients, they may bring up an interesting discussion point with a specialist. You would not want to use these promotionally, but memorizing th reference and date and key point made can be a good idea, to help you put a point you are making into perspective.

Now, you are ready to commence your project. Never assume you have all the answers, just keep trying to gather more information. Stay focused on the patient. Make up a sheet that shows logically what the advantages are of your competition as the staff at the clinic sees them. Add a column of offsetting points supported by clinical studies that you have studied. Plan a sequence of presentations that will hit the key points, stressing that the goal is *Patient Outcome.*

Your challenge at this point will be to engage a physician in a discussion of a specific patient type, and show in that instance, your product offers an advantage worth remembering. If the provider asks you to expand, you have the information that will be interesting to that doctor.

Take post-call notes so you know what your physicians said on each call, and, most importantly, what interested them.

After a couple of weeks, you return to the clinic, and are met with a comment about your product that is negative versus the competition. It is most likely a competitive representative has heard about your efforts and is trying to stop you.

You cannot be stopped if you stay focused on their patients and the published clinical studies. All you need to do is go to the clinical studies for both your product and your competitor's product, and build an approach that stops that comment. You can add a further approach to put the rep on the defensive. It never ceased to amaze us how some representatives would make bogus comments pulled out of thin air to protect their business. This is where preparation and notes will make your approach unstoppable.

Please visit our blog on www.sheeleyconsulting.com where we will discuss how to use a medical study to drive home a point in a stand-up 30-second presentation or sitting across from the provider at the desk. We will also provide insight into how to open a discussion about a medical journal article, and a whole lot more.

SAMPLE MEDICAL JOURNAL STUDY (REPRINT)
"THE UNITED STATES JOURNAL OF MEDICINE" (USJM)

We developed the *"United States Journal of Medicine"* medical journal study to demonstrate how we would dissect, interpret and analyze this study. Our analysis follows the study.

The comments we make in our analysis should apply to clinical studies in general. The USJM was also developed to give our readers who aren't familiar with journal articles an idea of all of the different parts of a srtudy look like---Abstract-Introduction-Materials & Methods- Results-Discussion-References.

Take time to answer the <u>Review Questions</u> following the journal study and the <u>two case</u> studies focusing on the *"US Journal of Medicine"* article and answer the questions related to each case.

Sample Reprint

THE UNITED STATES
JOURNAL OF MEDICINE

©Copyright, 2003, by Sheeley Consulting Group

Volume 9444   **January 33, 2003**   **Number 367**

VIRAL ELIMINATION IN HUMANS

R.W. Shoehorn, T.Anvil, V.Finesam, J.Huggs, and P.Spider

Abstract.   The purpose of the study was to determine whether humans infected with the DNA virus HSV-13 could have the virus removed from latency by therapy.   We studied 3,432 adults represented by 1,702 with infection and 1,730 with primary infections documented prior to entry in the placebo arm.   Infection was established by examining serum titers and by active culture of biopsy sites. All of the infected patients had active cultures after seven days of incubation at 37 degrees C, and their serum titers were positive for virus.   Patients were followed in a randomized, double blind trial of oral RCV for a mean of 36 months.   There was no initial difference in the treatment groups receiving the placebo or RCV. All the subjects in both treatment and placebo arms had ganglionic latency at the onset of the study. Recurrence rates in RCV treated patients were significantly reduced immediately following implementation of therapy. The placebo treated patients experienced recurrences that were similar to the treatment arm at onset, followed by a small drop in recurrences during the course of the study. (80% placebo subjects vs. 0% in RCV treated patients, ($p<0.0001$). These data suggest that when RCV is treatment is begun on HSV-13 infected individuals; the reduction of viral load and the reduction of the serum titer are significant.

P. Spider, MD, Department of Infectious Diseases, URCA School of Medicine, USA

Supported by a grant from the NIH, division of infectious diseases. All authors are free from financial support from the pharmaceutical industry. Drs. Shoehorn and Anvil are faculty members at DCU. Drs. Huggs and Spider are faculty members at URCA. Dr. Finesam is faculty at MacPhee.

INTRODUCTION

Herpes simplex Virus type 13 is an increasingly frequent primary and recurrent infection worldwide. Recurrence is common following the acute attack that causes additional morbidity and is responsible for spread of the disease. (1,2).

The introduction of antivirals such as RCV provides a major advance in therapy of recurrent disease (3,4). Oral RCV treatment has been shown to have significant effect on the shortening of the first episode of HSV-13, reducing both local and systemic symptoms. The recurrent infections have been treated with RCV with less success, as they are shorter in their clinical expression. There is evidence that prolonged treatment with RCV could reduce recurrence rate (5), so that clinicians did have the option to utilize RCV for each occurrence.

As part of a long-term prospective study of the natural history of HSV-13 we assessed the effects of treatment with RCV on both initial and recurrent infections in conjunction with a double blind trial of oral drug previously reported (6). This is a preliminary report of the data limited to the effects of RCV on recurrence patterns following HSV-13 infection over the first 3 years follow-up.

MATERIALS AND METHODS

Study population

Subjects with first episode HSV-13 infections with lesions present for <5 days were entered into a double blind, placebo controlled trial and randomized to receive either RCV or placebo, orally 5 mg Q.12h. for 7 days. The details and descriptions of these subjects have been previously reported (6). Subjects were then entered into the daily treatment phase comprised of daily RCV 2.5mg Q.D. or placebo for the duration of the study (36 months). All subjects were initially seen weekly, and categorized as having true primary infection if they had no serum titer within the first 14 days of the initial infection, and were culture positive at entrance to the study. All subjects later developed serum titers within the first 14 days of study. (Neutralizing antibody titer to HSV-13 <1:10 in serum and CSF negative in sera). Non-primary infections were not discovered during the trial in the active infection group. Patients with non-primary infections at onset of the trial were entered into the daily therapy arms, and randomized to drug or placebo. Non-primary infections are presented in Table I. Recurrence rates after first episode are shown in Table II. All patients were asked to report to the study clinical site whenever a recurrence was felt to be underway.

Follow up

Subjects were asked to return monthly once they were past their initial infection and had established a serum titer to HSV-13. Cultures were used to document infections when reported by patients. Subjects were sent e-mails monthly that requested updates on the status of recurrences (i.e. duration of lesions, systemic symptoms, and new lesions). Study coordinators routinely telephoned subjects if they failed to respond to the e-mails.

Statistical analysis

Groups were compared by Student's *t*-test analysis.

RESULTS

Population characteristics

Of the 3,432 patients (1,812 females and 1,620 males), who were entered into the original study from June 1999 to June 2002, 1,950 patients were available for follow up. There were 1,702 patients with HSV-13 primary infections, and an additional 78 who were found to have latent infections that were in the uninfected arm. Follow up took place from 24 to 36 months with a mean follow up period of 30 months. 91% of the subjects completed all 36 months of the trial. Two subjects dropped out of the study at two and three months, respectively, and were subsequently re-examined and found to have latent virus. A third patient dropped out at 6 weeks and was found to have no virus or titer when examined at two years. Patient then declined further medication. 735 patients were lost to follow up. No additional subjects were entered into the therapeutic trial or the placebo arm. None of subjects entered into the trial had recurrences after 18 months vs. 91% in the placebo arm.

Effects of RCV treatment in Non-primary HSV-13 infection

In Table 1, mean numbers of recurrences during each 6-month period are compared to each treatment arm: placebo or RCV. As illustrated, recurrence rates were significantly different between treatment groups, showing remarkable difference after 18 months.

Table I. Mean no. of recurrences 6 month

Length of follow up	Placebo	RCV	p-value *
0-6	77.2	69.1	<0.3
6-12	85.3	0.01	<0.0001
12-18	89.4	0.001	<0.0001
18-24	89.5	0.0	<0.00001
*Student t-test			

Effect of RCV treatment on recurrences following true primary HSV-13 infection

As shown in Table II, mean recurrence rates in RCV or placebo recipients are significantly significant during the first 6 months of follow up. After 6 months, recurrence rates in RCV treated subjects are significantly reduced when compared to placebo treated subjects, $p<0.01$. Recurrences dropped to virtually zero within the first 18 months of the study, in the treatment arm with RCV. The number of patients having recurrences in the placebo arm remained above 90% throughout the study. The relatively small drop of 9% in the placebo group was observed and noted.

Table II. Recurrence rates following first episode of true primary

HSV-13 infections

	Mean no. of recurrences		
Length of follow up	Placebo	RCV	p-value*
0-6	73.3	64.4	<0.3
6-12	83.3	0.0	<0.0001
12-18	85.5	0.0	<0.0001
18-24	86.5	0.0	<0.0001
*Student t-test			

Fig. 1.   Percentage of HSV-13 in treatment and placebo arms who continued to have recurrences over the 36 months of follow up.

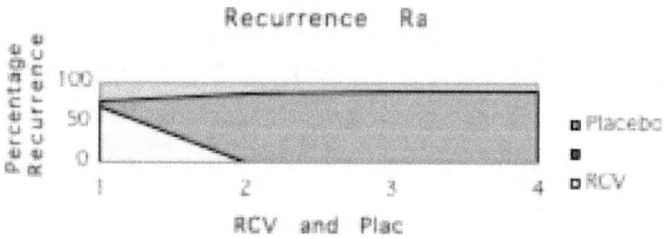

Adverse Events

After 36 months, 11.1% of the patients had adverse effects regardless of treatment group.

Table III lists adverse events with incidence of at least 1% documented in both placebo and drug group. Headache (3.1 vs. 2.0), and nausea (1.4 vs. 0.8) were statistically significant. Diarrhea, malaise, fever, upper respiratory infection (URI), while reported, did not demonstrate significant value.

Table III   Adverse events: placebo v. treatment

Event	Placebo	RCV	p-value*
Headache	2.0	3.1	0.052
Nausea	0.8	1.4	0.09
Diarrhea	1.7	1.3	0.5
Malaise	0.9	1.1	0.8
Fever	0.8	0.8	0.0
URI	0.4	0.5	0.0

*Student t-test

DISCUSSION

Our finding that RCV treatment affects the incidence, number, and duration of both titer positivity and recurrences (as confirmed by culture). Treatment with RCV 2.5mg Q.24h remained standard throughout the treatment arm, and similar placebo preparations were administered on the same schedule. This study further demonstrated that while initial treatment with RCV did not affect long-term outcome of the patients' recurrence pattern, a daily, low-dose administration of RCV was able to clear the infections.

The numbers of subjects experiencing recurrences were significantly reduced in RCV recipients vs. placebo recipients within 6 months ($p<0.0001$). Laboratory tests, neutralizing antibody titer and/or direct swab viral culture, conclusively demonstrate that in this treatment group, latent infection did not persist. Placebo arm did report a persistence of both the neutralizing antibody titer and positive cultures obtained from lesion sites reported during clinic visits. We were not able to obtain biopsies of ganglia to verify the presence or absence of latent virus due to the invasive and costly nature of these procedures.

The natural history of RCV infections has not demonstrated any great number of spontaneous resolutions or disappearances of virus over time in humans. There is evidence in animal models that therapy with antivirals with a similar mode of action can be effective on specifically sensitive viral strains. The elimination of titer demonstrated in this study, combined with the complete lack of recurrent infections, lends itself to the premise that the HSV-13 viral particles continually replicate to some degree wherever they are in the host organism. This low level of activity renders them susceptible to inhibition and elimination by RSV. Further observations confirming elimination of viral antigen presence and absence of recurrent disease during the trial in the treatment arm would tend to confirm our hypothesis. However, the mechanism of causation of recurrent infections remains unconfirmed and unknown, despite sufficient patient numbers in the study to record any pattern of stimulus causing recurrence. Our patient follow up (over 79%) was high for studies of this nature, and deserve some further note regarding utilization of new technologies, specifically the internet and electronic mail to assist in patient communications.

CONCLUSION

The results of this study represent careful follow-up of a significant patient cohort, and demonstrate clearly the safety and efficacy of RCV and its impact on the history of HSV-13 infections. Both primary and non-primary patients showed reduction in both recurrence and serum positivity. Further, despite the length of therapy, it is important to note that adverse events were not the primary reason for drop out or inability to complete the study, in either group. Our previously published observations (6) together with these findings represent a comprehensive view of the natural experiences both patients with acute infections and recurrent HSV-13 infections. We believe this is due the *in vitro* observation that HSV-13 is exquisitely sensitive to RCV when the agent is present at low concentrations over a prolonged length of time. Further studies to determine optimal dosing of RCV in this population and minimal patient/drug exposure time should be explored.

REFERENCES

1. Herman A, Whitstaf B, Anvil T, Initial and recurring infections of HSV-13. *Ann Inf Med* 143: 958-972, 1998.

2. Whitstaf B, Finesam V, Prevalence and symptoms of HSV-13 in adults. *J Crinil Data* 12: 111-131, 1997.

3. Fogeldurg D, Prince R, RCV therapy for systemic HSV-13. *Arche Detramat* 194: 7-13, 1996.

4. Fogeldurg D, Prince R, RCV effect on acute HSV-13 infections in humans. *J Inflect Dis* 1: 5-11, 1996.

5. Imming R, Cessation of recurrences in three patients treated with RCV. *J Scandish Oft.* 12: 97, 1997.

6. Shoehorn R, Anvil T, Finesam V, Huggs J, Spider P, Oral therapy for initial and recurrent HSV-13. *Arch Patient Dis* 11: 124-130, 2001.

HOW WE WOULD APPROACH DISSECTING & ANALYZING
"THE US JOURNAL OF MEDICINE" (USJM)

Authors

Where was the study done? *This study indicates 3-study sites, and the data is not broken down by study site.* More than one study site (if more than one, be watchful to see how carefully each site has aligned their testing, randomization and therapy). *No comments in our USJM study.* Did the authors have any financial interest in the study outcome? None in this USJM study. Are they paid speakers presenting this study to various medical groups? *None noted.*

Abstract

Often readers do not have time to go beyond this overview. It can yield some insight into questions about study organization, size, analysis and reporting. Often a date of journal submission is listed. *This journal did not list submission dates.* If there is a significant pause in time between the datre and the date of the journal publication, ask yourself why? *How many times did they have to resubmit?*

If there are very few patients studied, the outcomes shift to the <u>anecdotal</u> category requiring formal blinded study.

What was the study designed to analyze? Is this data going to be helpful to improve selected patient outcomes with new insight? In other words, are the results valuable for your patient outcomes? HSV-13 is contagious and is spreading worldwide. It will be important to most practices. How many patients were entered, and how many completed the study? *3,432 entered and we will have to read further to see how many completed the study. This is a relatively large study, and the testing proves strong confidence.*

Introduction

This is an overview. Medical Center patients are more complex since they have been referred from the community, and thus patient analysis may show different aspects of <u>incidence</u> and <u>prevalence</u> from your community practice patients. Bottom line is to answer the question, *"How might this study change the way my patients are treated and tested?"* The drug 'RCV' has two oral formulations, 5mg Q. 12h and 2.5mg Q. 24h. These are simple regimens, usually with high compliance.

Ask what limitations were placed upon the study patients testing and treatment that might not apply to the patients you see and treat. *Community based practices cannot afford to see patients monthly, for example.* Often medical center tests are not covered by community patient insurance plans.

Materials & Methods

These allow authors to determine cutoff points and acceptable ranges of results that will vary from those available to the community practices, and also allow the authors to choose 'windows of analysis' for p-values. *This study sates a p-value that is very nice, p<0.0001.*

Results

The population characteristics are worth looking into. Particularly check to see starting population size versus those completing the study. *Begin with 3,492, followed up with a reduced population of 1,950. Why did those 1,542 patients not stay with the study?* Were they eliminated by the authors, if so, where is the analysis of thos patients? They may have had characteristics that would have decreased p-value, or they may have had other aspects found during work-up that necessitated their removal. *All of these should have been noted in the study to enhance credibility.*

Adverse Effects

There may have been reasons for discontinung a small group of patients, and *you want to know what thos findings were.*

Discussion

Look for insights here that may provide reason to change your patient testing or treatment if they are strong enough factors.

Patient follow-up? How much effort was expended in contacting those patients who did not report for their clinic visits? This is an area to focus upon, and insight gained from your patient population may help you understand some of these aspects.

Conclusion

This is a good place to visit-it usually asks for further studies, of course. Aside from that constant, this section should place the study findings into perspective about how these authors regard the placement and value of their results. Ask, 'does this apply to my patients, or is there a patient I know of who could benefit from these insights?'

References

There is only one other study cited. *Is that because this is a relatively new infection? Or did they eliminate some references for some reason. Were many of them by the same author?*

H'm. Read through the references to see what other studies the author looked at, what publication dates were, and ask yourself if there are perhaps a couple of studies you want to request and study for your patients.

Closing Observations

This US Journal of Medicine study was basically good, with a large group of patients and laboratory testing. Could it have been better with more useful information? Absolutely. And now you can see see how to appraise other clinical studies

Sample Reprint "The United States Journal of Medicine", vol 9444, January 33, 2003, No 367, *"Viral Elimination In Humans"*

Briefing Guide©

Answers to the questions asked in the "Briefing Guide"© are shown for *"The US Journal of Medcine"* at the end.

US JOURNAL OF MEDICINE---REVIEW QUESTIONS:

1. In the Introduction, the authors write of the problems with RCV in treating recurrent infections, They state:

    A. There are no recurrent infections after an initial treatment with RCV

    B. There was no difference between RCV in initial treatments and recurrent treatment

    C. The recurrent infections have been treated with RCV with less success as they are shorter in their clinical expression

2. Patients were allowed in to the initial treatment arm if they had been:

    A. Subjects with firt episode HSV-13 infections with lesions present for <5-days

    B. Subjects with either recurrent or first episode HSV-13

    C. Subjects with first episode HSV-13 with lesions present for >5 dys

3. Dosing for the initial treatment infections was:

    A. 5 mg. Q 12 hours for 7 days

    B. 5 mg. Q 8 hours for 7 days

    C. 5mg Q 12 hours for 10 days

4. Patients with non-primary infections were enrolled:

    A. In short term therapy arm

    B. In daily treatment arm

    C. Given a choice between a short-term therapy arm and daily treatment

5. Patients with primary infections were asked to return to monitored serum titers:

    A. At one month

    B. At two months

    C. Weekly

6. Of the original 3,422 patients enrolled, how many were followed?

    A. 1,950

    B. 3,000

    C. 1,450

7. The follow up period was:

    A. Between 24 and 36 months with an average of 30

    B. Between 12 and 36 months with an average of 24

    C. Between 24 and 48 month with an average of 30

8. What was the percentage who completed 36 months?

    A. 78%

    B. 91%

    C. 45%

9. The mean number of recurrence at 6-months following non-primary infections:

    A. 85.3

    B. 90.0

    C. 88.9

10. The mean number of recurrence at 18-24 mnths following primary infections

    A. 86.5

    B. 91.0

    C. 75.8

11. Test used to confirm results were by:

    A. Western blot test

    B. Neutralizing antibody titers as well as the direct swab viral culture

    C. Bacterial cultures

Answers: 1=C; 2=A; 3=A; 4=B; 5=C; 6=A; 7=A; 8=B; 9=A; 10=A; 11=B

CASE STUDIES USING:

"UNITED STATES JOURNAL OF MEDICINE"

Viral Eliminations In Humans

Instructions: using the *US Journal of Medicine* study, first read *"The Case"* and then answer the questions listed under *"The Representative"*

CASE STUDY # 1...TWO HIGH-PRESCRIBING FAMILY PRACTICE PROVIDERD

The Case

You conduct a lunch-n-learn with two high-prescribing Family Practice providers.

Dr Smith uses RCV for short-term therapy but he does not believe in long-term therapy. Dr Jones uses RCV only for initial infections, but does not see it being very effective for RCV for recurrent infections.

Dr Smith is an extrovert and Dr Jones is very quiet and spends most of the lunch doing paper work. He will give you a minute at most.

Your call objective---to get Dr Smith and Dr Jones' commitment to use RCV long term.

The Representative

Using the United States Journal of Medicine study:

What opening statement can you use with both Dr Jones and Dr Smith if they are in the room together?

Which part of the "*Materials and Methods*" would prove useful?

How would you use the results to support your conclusion?

Prepare a 30-second detail for Dr Jones

Discuss how to bridge to the next product or paper after presentation of this one

How would you use the *"Result"?*

CASE STUDY # 2

The Case

Dr Alan Paul uses RCV for acute cases but never used it for suppressive therapy of recurrent therapy. In the past, he has feared resistance and lack of efficacy with use of long-term therapy. Dr Paul is difficult to see and rarely sees sales representatives. You are putting your samples in the sample cabinet and Dr Paul walks up to look for a sample.

The Representative

Using The United States Journal of Medicine

Based on The *"Abstract"*how would you open a discussion with Dr Paul?

Based on The "Abstract", design a 30-sec presentation by the sample cabinet

What can you use in the *"Abstract"* to show efficacy for long-term therapy?

How many patients completed the study and what is the benefit to Dr Paul?

You have Dr Paul's interest, use the charts in the *"Results"* section for a support statement on RCV efficacy for suppression therapy

"if you don't throw it, they can't hit it" -- Lefty Gomez

UNITED STATES JOURNAL OF MEDICINE (USJM)©

"VIRAL ELIMINATION IN HUMANS"
January 33, 2013, vol 9444, Number 367

HOW WE WOULD <u>PRESENT</u> THIS STUDY (USJM) AT A GRAND ROUNDS PRESENTATION OR A JOURNAL CLUB:

The *"US Journal of Medicine"* (included with your manual) was put together and written by us to have a study we could use as an example to show our readers how the different sections of a study are listed in a study---authors, abstract, introduction, Material & Method, Results, Discussion and References---and, for our purpose, to provide you with an example of how we would present this study at a Grand Rounds meeting or Journal Club.

Preparation

1. Do a literature search of "Human, HSV-13, Latency to see what has been published on the subject to date.

2. Check with your laboratory to see how they identify HSV-13 infections, whether by serum titer analysis or growth from culture swabs.

3. Find out how rapidly results can be reported, knowing that positive results are quicker than growing a negative culture

4. Find out how many HSV-13 infections they have identified to date from the medical center patients. If you can identify presenting aspects of these patients, that data would provide strong interest from the staff.

5. Ask clinical PharmD for pharmacologic aspects of treatment with antivirals, including HCV utilized in this study.

6. Following your short preparation on HSV-13, you have found that there is only one treatment mentions, and that this is the second clinical study done on patients identified with this virus.

7. Further, you found that your lab does not routinely do cultures for HSV-13, and after your preparation to the Staff, a committee can decide whether to add this virus on the laboratory listing of cultures and titers that include HSV-13.

PREPARATION OF THE STUDY

The Abstract

- This study was supported by a grant from the NIH_

- The purpose of the study to determine whether humans infected with the DNA virus HSV-13 could have the virus eliminated prior to latency in acute cases, as well as how treatment modified recurrence rates

- The study 'n' number was 3,432 adult patients, with 1,702 having the latent infection and 1,730 with primary infections. These were identified with culture of sites and serum titers to differentiate primary infections from established latency. Random allocation placed patients in either the treatment are or the placebo arm.

- Recurrence rates were significantly reduced with initiation of therapy, with the placebo group experiencing continued recurrences with a p-value of $p<0.0001$.

- Significantly, treatment with RCV yielded a 0% recurrence rate in the treatment group.

- Herpesvirus group infections yield ganglionic latency and a re associated with the contagious spread and the potential for a small group of cancers over time.

Introduction:

- HSV is increasingly frequent worldwide infection with both primary and recurrent aspects.

- Early identification and treatment reduce the establishment of latency

- The question of prolonged therapeutic treatment versus serial treatment of each recurrence has not been studied to date.

- The study followed the recurrence pattern of patients for a total of 3-years.

Materials and Methods:

- Patients with first episode HSV-13 and lesions present for less than 5-days were entered into the trial utilizing RCV 5 mg Q. 12h. for 7 days

- If there was no serum titer within 14 days, the patients randomized to therapy received RCV 2.5 mg Q.D. or placebo the duration of the 36-month study.

- True primary infections demonstrated no serum titer within 14 days of initial infection, and were culture positive at study entry

- Patients were asked to report to the clinical site when a recurrence was felt.

- Subjects returned monthly once past their initial infection if they had established a serum titer to HSV-13,

- Cultures were used to document infections.

The Results:

- Of the initial 3,492 patients entered into the study, 1,950 were available for follow-up.

- Of those patients, 1,702 had primary HSV-13 infections, while 78 were found to have latent infections to the uninfected arm.

- The mean follow-up was 30-months

- 735 patients were lost to follow-up.

- Significantly, none of the subjects entered into the treatment arm had recurrences after 18-mpnths versus 91% in the placebo arm

- Show overhead of Table II and Figure 1 to demonstrate recurrence rate numbers and percentage of recurrence.

- Table III lists adverse effects, placebo versus treatment

Discussion:

- Key Finding---long term low dose preventative therapy was able to clear the infections.

- The placebo arm did not demonstrate spontaneous resolution or disappearance of virus during the 36-month study.

- Studied patient follow-up was high for studies of this nature at 79%

Conclusion:

This study demonstrated efficacy of RCV and that therapy was effective in reducing infections with a low percentage of adverse effects. *In vitro* the virus HSV-13 is sensitive to RCV

"The greatest gift one person can give another is time" --Anonymous

SAMPLE DETAILS

FIRST ENCOUNTER

The detail takes place in the infectious disease department library. This physician has not been seen before by anyone from the company, and is now entering a critically important specialty.

The plan for the call is that at the end of the call, the physician will be focused on the value of identifying the virus (HIV-13) and offer RCV to either patients with initial infections or to those that he encounters with recurrent infections.

Rep: Dr. Newby, Hello! I am Del Vinlit from Acme Pharmaceuticals. The subject that would be most interesting to you right now, as well as most helpful for many patients is HIV-13 an effective treatment specifically for those patients who suffer from either initial or recurrent outbreaks. Have you seen many of these outbreaks?

Dr. Newby: A fair number, yes.

Rep: Yes, they are tough for the patients to work through and the lesions are so contagious aren't they?

Dr Newby: Yes, that's how it is spread.

Rep: How do you make the differential diagnosis?

Dr. Newby: Once my differential diagnosis includes HIV-13, I will order either a culture if it is a primary infection, or a first outbreak, or a serum titer if it is a recurrent infection.

Rep: That's great! You have the best tools at hand when you use cultures or titers.

Rep: Dr. Newby, earlier this year, Dr Shoehorn, et al published a study that demonstrated a remarkable effect on HSV-13 patients. They studied 3,432 patients and were able to follow up with 1,950 at the end of the study interval. Their goal was to measure response following six months of daily therapy following both initial and recurrent infections (Rep shows first paragraph of US JM article).

Dr Newby: Was the study blinded and placebo-controlled?

Rep: Yes, the design was double blind, placebo-controlled with patient-initiated follow up for outbreaks.

            (Indicates the point of the Study Population that states that "All subjects later developed serum titers within the first 14-days of study" and "All patients were asked to report to their clinical site whenever a recurrence was felt to be underway".

Rep: Further, the study used frequent e-mail follow up with clinical RN's to assure compliance and maximum collection of data through the duration of the study. Here it is on page 2 of the Materials & Methods section:

            (Indicates the e-mail part under the Follow-Up Section: "Subjects were sent e-mails monthly regarding recurrences".

Dr. Newby: That is a well-thought-out approach. Were the results significant?

Rep: That is the best part, Dr Newby. The comparison between placebo and RCV 2.5mg Q.D. not only showed a p-value of <0.0001, but also demonstrated viral elimination by the end of the trial.

            (Indicates "Effects of RCV treatment on recurrences" section that states "Recurrences dropped to virtually zero within the first 18-months of the study in the treatment arm with RCV").

Dr Newby: Did the treatment arm patients retain their viral titers?

Rep: Good question. No. titers dropped to zero, further documenting the elimination of the virus particles as antigens in the patients

(Shows: paragraph under figure one that states, "The tests that were used, including both the neutralizing antibody titer as well as the direct swab viral culture conclusively demonstrate that in this study population, the latent infection did not persist").

Dr Newby: This approach is one that will be helpful to infected patients, and I am not sure of such success with anything for other members of the HSV family.

Rep: That is true, Dr. Newby. RCV 2.5mg QD for 6-months represents a truly large gain in your ability to offer patients improved quality of life and reduction in viral load. Don't you agree that this is an approach worth remembering?

Dr Newby: Yes, I will remember this.

Rep: Dr. Newby, what works best for you? Will you enter RCV 2.5mg Q.D. in your PDA in the HSV-13 section or will some other method work for you?

Dr. Newby: Actually, that is a good idea. I will enter RCV now in my new PDA. Also, I'd like a small packet of patient information fliers to give to my patients.

Rep: Would that be best in the ID clinic, with the nurse, or in the ID office?

Dr Newby: If you can do both that would cover most of the bases.

Rep: Thanks for discussing HSV-13 therapy with RCV. I look forward to bringing you brief updates as they come out. If you have any questions or need a response from our Medical Department, here is my card with a number you can out in your PDA as well.

Dr Newby: Thanks. I'll do that. I appreciate your being brief and to the point. Nice to see something with real value for a change.

Rep: You're welcome. I look forward to working with you.

Discussion

What did this representative do in a critical situation? This is a new customer and a credible relationship will be key.

- A brief description of the paper and results was presented in a manner that established a patient-centered window for conversation.

- A probe was used to focus on the patient aspect of the paper and to allow you to make the conversation beneficial to you both. What if Dr Newby had NOT encountered these patients in his past experience? Then you would need to be prepared to take a different route through the paper. If you hadn't probed and sallied forth, you would have lost a great opportunity.

- The focus on patient benefits of RCV therapy was reinforced with facts and a process that makes scientific sense. In the United States J of Medicine article, the specific patient types are patients with initial infections and patients with recurrent infections. That is whom Dr Newby should consider for therapy.

- The slam-dunk of showing valid trial results with drug at recommended doses "the comparison between placebo and RCV 2.5mg Q.D. not only showed a p-value of <0.0001, but also demonstrated viral elimination by the end of the trial". At this point, if a physician has time, he is going to ask a question. If the physician doesn't, thank him for his time and ask him if he would use RCV for HIV-13 infected patients, mentioning the prescribing information.

30-SECOND STAND UP

You have met Dr. Hamby in the hallway. You have now 30 seconds for your detail. You keep the reprint in your bag and have the Doctor sign your signature card.

Rep: Doctor, nice to see you. Thanks for signing for samples. Because we have discussed the number of patients you see with HSV-13, I thought you might be interested in a recent study from the United States Journal of Medicine, Dr. Hamby. In is a double blind, placebo-controlled study RCV to reduced viral titers to 0% when patients were kept on once-a-day suppressive regimen.

Dr. Hamby: O.K.

Rep: (Takes the reprint out of bag): Doctor, here's the study. Dr. Shoehorn and his colleagues independently demonstrated RCV efficacy reduces viral titers to zero after 18 months of therapy.

Dr. Hamby: O.K.

Rep: The benefit for your patients is that with a one Q.D. dosing at 2.5 mg, (how prescriptions for once a day are written) viral infections are really cleared. This will give your patients back control of their lives---they will be infection free.

Dr. Hamby: Thanks. Leave a copy and I'll see if I can take a look at it.

Rep: Will do. I think you will find the paper rather interesting and with great clinical relevance. I would like to get your 'read' on it. How about getting together about the study next Thursday, after the Journal Club, while you head for rounds?

Dr. Hamby: Sounds good. See you then.

Rep: Great. Thanks for your time.

Discussion

What was accomplished in the 30-second detail to Dr. Hamby?

- Dr. Hamby is aware that you pay attention to his practice and what is important to him---you know that he sees HIV-13 patients.

- You reinforced the prescribing habit of RCV by demonstrating its efficacy in another use. If you knew Dr. Hamby was also using a competitive product to treat HSV-13, you would want to include a specific patient subtype in your opening remarks. Instead of the opening "because of the number of patients you see with HSV-13", if Dr. Hamby were using a competitor's product, you would want to zero in on a specific type of patient where your product has an advantage.

- You didn't let Dr. Hamby's comment of "OK" throw you. He is listening to what you say to see if you are presenting information that will be of value to him. If it makes you more comfortable, you should acknowledge the "OK", and carry on.

- You have demonstrated the credibility of your product and your information by pointing out that the study was independent. Even if Dr. Hamby does not read the article, he will remember that the results are credible. This demonstrates you are a valuable and reliable source of information

BRIEFING GUIDE©

Purpose: This guide is a tool that will allow you to create a "brief" for journal articles you are using. It will assist you as you set forth your plan, and should be kept with a copy of the reprint. Even when you are comfortable with using reprints, you may find this tool useful as a reminder or "mental checklist". The second page allows you to determine with whom you should plan to use the reprint in your next call cycle.

1.   What is the title of the paper and its publication source?

2.   Authors. Where do the primary authors practice? What is/re. The author's primary affili-ation(s)?

Author	Institution/Practice

3.   Abstract or Summary Overview.
     What was the purpose, and what was the final outcome of the study?

4.   Sponsorship/bias. Where did the financial support from the paper originate?
     Pharmaceutical company? Other funding?   Or what are the disclosures with regard to funding and/or affiliations?

5. Study Design. What was the study design?_____

    a. Was the study double-blinded? _

        1. Was there a control or placebo arm? _____

        2. What method of statistical analysis was used? _____

    b. Patient Inclusion

        1. How many patients were entered into the study? _____ _____

        2. What types of patients were studied? _____

        3. How were the patients selected? _____

        4. What is (are) the marketed/approved dose(s) of the drug? _____

    c. Product/Tests Studied

        1. What doses of drugs were studied? _____

    d. What relevant laboratory tests were used? _____

6. Figures, Tables. Which figures and tables are helpful? _____

    What can they demonstrate to your customer?

7. Safety.

    a. What are the overall safety findings? _____

    b. How do they compare to historical (other) trials? _____

    c. What are the significant SAE's? (Significant adverse event) _____

        1.How do these compare within treatment groups? _____

    d. Was the number (n) of patients large enough to determine if these adverse events were a fair representation/statistically significant?

    e. Did the adverse events improve when the drugs were discontinued?

8. Patient Outcomes.

    What kind of patients had the best outcomes? _____

What kind of patients had the worst outcomes? __

Describe any equivocal findings/outcomes: _____

9. What is the clinical relevance of this paper, or how will it impact everyday practice?

9a. Describe, in one sentence, the value this study brings to/for your product.

10. Who on your call sheet will benefit from knowing this information (today/this week/this cycle) and why?

Customer	Main Point to Discuss – or main point of persuasion – e.g. author, institution, statistical power, patient type etc.

BRIEFING GUIDE

P<u>urpose:</u> This is how we would complete the Briefing Guide for the United States Journal of Medicine, "Viral Elimination In Humans".

1. What are the title of the paper and its publication source? _Title=Viral Elimination in Humans; Published in The United States Journal of Medicine, Vol. 9444, Jan 33, 2003, No. 367._

2. Authors. Where do the primary authors practice? What is/re. the author's primary affiliation(s)

Author	Institution/Practice
R.W.Shoehorn	_DCU faculty_
T. Anvil	_DCU faculty_
V.Finesam	_MacPhee faculty_

3. Abstract or Summary Overview.

    What was the purpose, and what was the final outcome of the study? _Purpose: To determine if HSV-13 virus can be removed from latency by suppressive therapy. Outcome: Recurrence rates in RCV treated patients were reduced immediately._

4. Sponsorship/bias. Where did the financial support from the paper originate?

Pharmaceutical company? Other funding? Or what are the disclosures with regard to funding and/or affiliations? *Study funded by NIH grand, Div. of Infect. Dis.; No pharmaceutical company backing. Therefore, minimal bias.*

5. Study Design. What was the study design? *Double Blind Placebo Controlled.*

   a. Was the study double-blinded? *Yes, it was.*

      1. Was there a control or placebo arm? *Yes, there was.*

      2. What method of statistical analysis was used? *Student's t-test*

   b. Patient Inclusion

      1. How many patients were entered into the study? *3,432 patients enrolled.*

      2. What types of patients were studied? *Pnts w/ initial or recurrent HSV-13*

      3. How were the patients selected? *Examination, viral culture and serum titer tests.*

      4. What is (are) the marketed/approved dose(s) of the drug? *RCV 2.5 mg. Q 24h.*

   c. Product/Tests Studied

      1. What doses of drugs were studied? *2.5 mg. tabs*

   d. What relevant laboratory tests were used? *Viral serum titer/viral cultures.*

6. Figures, Tables. Which figures and tables are helpful? *Fig. I, Tables I, II, & III.*

   What can they demonstrate to your customer?

7. Safety.

   a. What are the overall safety findings? *Minimal Hedache, Nausea.*

   b. How do they compare to historical (other) trials? *Less than higher dose episodic treatment.*

   c. What are the significant SAE's? (significant adverse event) *Headache and Nausea had borderline statistical significance.*

      1. How do these compare within treatment groups? *All similar.*

   d. Was the number (n) of patients large enough to determine if these adverse events were a fair representation/statistically significant? *Yes, it was.*

e. Did the adverse events improve when the drugs were discontinued? *Not known.*

8. Patient Outcomes.

   What kind of patients had the best outcomes? *Those with frequent recurrences.* What kind of patients had the worst outcomes? *Infrequent recurrences harder to measure changes.*

   Describe any equivocal findings/outcomes:*None noted during study.*

9. What is the clinical relevance of this paper, or how will it impact everyday practice? *Documents suppression as a very effective way to treat HSV-13*

9a. Describe, in one sentence, the value this study brings to/for your product.

   Proves daily suppression as strongest way for patient/physician to treat HSV-13.

10. Who on your call sheet will benefit from knowing this information (today/this week/this cycle) and why?

Customer	Main Point to Discuss – or main point of persuasion – eg author, institution, statistical power, patient type etc.
Dr. Kline	Episodic proven; offer suppression next
Dr. MacQuist	Abstract – show efficacy vs. side efx
Dr,. O'Malia	
Dr. Start	
Dr. Whisnant	
Dr. Quinn	
Dr. Levy	
Dr. Post	
Dr. Orr	

WHO WE ARE

We started out in territories selling around 100 products (everything in the Burroughs Wellcome Co---now Glaxo Smith Kline---Catalog), while studying every night and taking tests to certify on all product groups during the first year. Passing was 90 and each one had to be passed. We had drugs for Oncology, anesthesia, Infectious Disease, and most other specialties. Many of them were sold in several areas of our hospitals that we visited regularly. That start gave us a very broad range of experience! We later taught all of the levels of representative courses in HQ, giving us teaching experience. Both of us were promoted to hospital sales. What we learned and shared across the country taught us vocabularies and gave insights into key specialties that we continually modified and improved. Our writings are the result of two guys paying attention with a very steep learning curve. We gained acceptance to attend virtually all of the daily, weekly, and monthly specialty conferences, grand rounds, even M&M's. A few other competitive reps gained acceptance and mostly they were interested only in mentions of their products. Seeing a bigger picture, we exchanged many aspects of how residents learn over the years. What we learned is written here as a gift to you. It will save you time, enhance your approach, and increase both your rapport and sales as you earn acceptance with many patient treatment teams. Attaining these 'memberships' is quite a leap beyond what most reps attain. We became experts in developing relationships with key thought leaders. We know it will take hard work, confident that our approach will enhance your daily contact with professionals in medicine while providing improved outcomes for countless specific patients. There is no similar modification of approach that we are aware of in the medical sales marketplace.

THE END...

It is not important whether you sell pharmaceutical products or artificial knees as a medical equip-ment representative, the road to success in both fields is paved with knowledge of your product and knowing your product's competition. We can't emphasize this enough.

Every top performing representative we ever supervised, whether calling on providers in their private offices or in a teaching medical center, shared one thing in common---a high level of knowledge about their product and a higher level (it seemed) of their competitor's product. As one Representative said to me years ago, *"Product knowledge. There is no substitute"*.

It took us a long time to move past the *"tell-tll-tell-close"* sales presentation we first learned in taking the week-long Xerox Professional Sales Skills course. *"Doctor, would you please use Septra on your next five patients who have a urinary tract infection?"* It is painful to even remember the Xerox course to this day. It took us a long time sitting in Grand Rounds presentations, Journal Club meetings and M&M conferences to learn how doctors think, make drug selection decisions and get a provider to use our drug for the very first time.

You goal is to be viewed as a consultant by the providers you call on. At this level there isn't a competitor out there that can beat you.

Don't forget to look at the review questions, 2-case studies and how we would dissect and analyze the study at the end of the ***"United States Journal Of Medicine"*** journal article we wrote for this book..

Please visit our website www.sheeleyconsulting.com. If you have any questions or comments about this book, let us hear from you.

Ron Sheeley: Rsheeley09@gmail.com

Paul Snyder: Psnyder1@indyrr.com